EVERYDAY
ESSENTIAL OILS

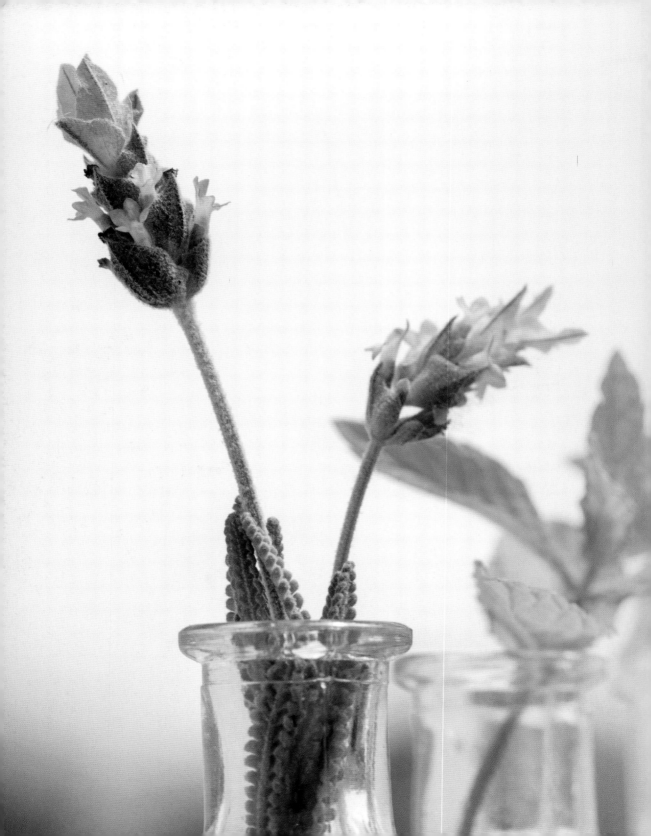

DANIÈLE FESTY

EVERYDAY ESSENTIAL OILS

300 BRILLIANT REASONS TO USE ESSENTIAL OILS EVERY DAY

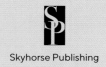

Skyhorse Publishing

This edition first published by Eddison Books Limited

First Skyhorse Publishing Edition 2019

Skyhorse Publishing books may be purchased in bulk at special discounts for
sales promotion, corporate gifts, fund-raising, or educational purposes. Special
editions can also be created to specifications. For details, contact the Special
Sales Department, Skyhorse Publishing, 307 West 36th Street, 11th Floor,
New York, NY 10018 or info@skyhorsepublishing.com.

Skyhorse® and Skyhorse Publishing® are registered trademarks
of Skyhorse Publishing, Inc.®, a Delaware corporation.

Visit our website at www.skyhorsepublishing.com.

10 9 8 7 6 5 4 3 2 1

Library of Congress Cataloging-in-Publication data is available on file.

Cover design by Fogdog Creative

ISBN: 978-1-63158-430-5
eISBN: 978-1-63158-439-8

Printed in China

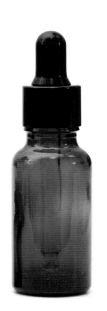

First published in France in 2017 by Leduc.s Éditions as
Les 6 Huiles Essentielles Indispensables

PLEASE NOTE
The author and publisher cannot accept any responsibility for misadventure
resulting from the practice of any of the principles and techniques set out in this
book. This book is not intended as guidance for the treatment of serious health
problems; please take note of any cautionary advice given, and refer to a medical
professional if you are in any doubt about any aspect of your condition.

CONTENTS

INTRODUCTION

Fragrant essential oils work gently but surely. For a long time, they were the exclusive province of perfumers and played a somewhat anonymous role in the manufacture of cosmetics. More recently, they've come out of the wings to take centre stage, reminding us how to look after ourselves safely and effectively.

Here, in this book, we unveil the real stars. Here are six essential oils, which excel on every front; they're all top performers, versatile and unique. The effective, natural properties of these six superstars will enhance your everyday life. Each one has its own special qualities, its primary and secondary roles, but all serve the same purpose – to look after us, to beautify, and to make day-to-day life that bit smoother and more pleasant. The six are: tea tree oil, lemon, lavender, peppermint, and damask rose.

In these pages, you'll discover 300 great ways to use these essential oils. Their potent qualities make them effective everywhere – for beauty care, safeguarding your health, or looking after your home or garden. Everyone can benefit. You want to get back into shape? They can help in slimming self-massage oils that encourage your body to eliminate toxins and waste, helping you to dislodge stored fat (see page 34). Whether you're fifteen, twenty, thirty, forty, fifty, sixty, or older, you'll find an essential oil cosmetic programme tailor-made for you, with scrubs, masks, toners, makeup removers, lip balms, and more.

The oils are also on hand to help you treat daily cuts and grazes safely and effectively. For a cut, use 2 drops of the most antiseptic essential oils (see page 90). For head lice, there's a remedy that kills off the eggs (see page 93). Or perhaps it's insomnia, toothache, or pregnancy pains – you'll find solutions for so many different conditions and diseases.

Another great use of essential oils is in the home, as an alternative to polluting cleaning chemicals. Get rid of grease from surfaces with 'Miracle' homemade products (see 'Miracle' grease remover, page 100). Banish the food bugs that squat in cupboards (see page 102), and keep your pet's coat glossy and parasite-free (see page 123).

Here, however, we won't tell you all the 300 good reasons for introducing essential oils into your life; you can discover them in the following pages.

CHOOSE QUALITY PRODUCTS

Forget market stalls or convenience stores: you shouldn't stint on quality when it comes to essential oils. In a pharmacy or shop that sells natural or organic products, you have every chance of finding good products, and perhaps, good advice as well. The bottle should be coloured (brown or green, for instance) to preserve the properties of the essential oils, which are sensitive to UV rays. If the bottle has a dropper, all the better, as the drop is the basic unit of measurement in aromatherapy and in the essential oil applications in this book.

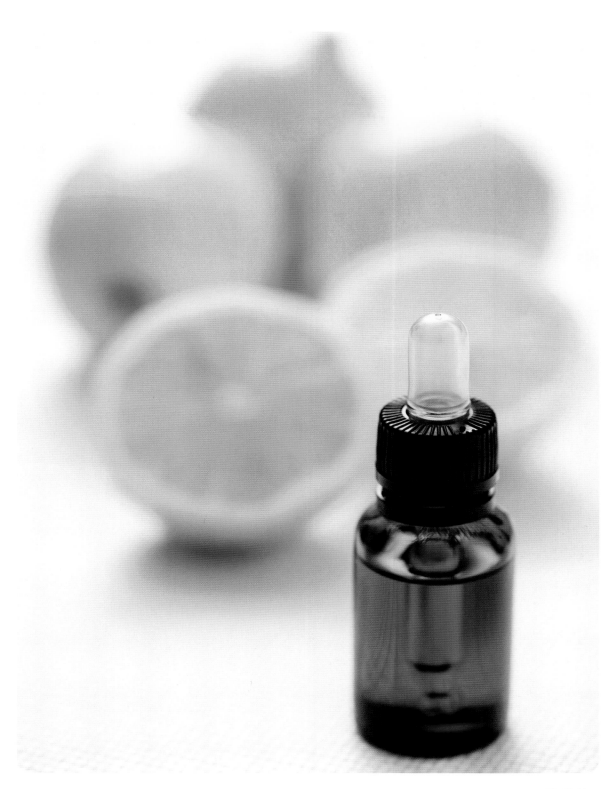

As a minimum, the label should mention the common name of the plant (such as lavender), its scientific species name (in this example, *Lavendula angustifolia*), the details of the supplier, the batch number, the part of the plant used (for lavender, the flower), the name of its most prominent biochemical constituent (in this case linalol), a mention of its therapeutic grade, and its expiry date.

TAKE CARE WHEN USING THEM

Essential oils can be enjoyed in a host of ways – in herbal teas, baths, rubs, massages, inhalations, in saunas, or diffused into the air. However, whichever application you choose, whether ingesting or applying an essential oil, the amounts to be used are very precisely stipulated. Never guess or improvise; essential oils are fragrant little treasures, but only if you use them carefully and in moderation.

CONTRAINDICATIONS AND PRECAUTIONS

- Never increase the recommended amounts.
- Do not swallow essential oils in their pure form (except, perhaps, in rare cases, a drop of peppermint or lemon). They should only be ingested following expert advice and precisely as stipulated, and diluted in a carrier substance, such as olive oil or honey.
- With a very few exceptions (lavender and tea tree essential oils, applied to very small areas), do not use pure essential oils directly on your skin. They should first be diluted in a carrier oil, such as sweet almond, macadamia, or jojoba.
- Pregnant women should be extremely cautious. If you use the oils on your skin, do so sparingly and for no more than three or four days in a row. Avoid ingesting any essential oils during pregnancy, except – perhaps – lemon or ginger, which can help combat morning sickness in the first month.
  * If pregnant, always consult a qualified aromatherapist first.
- If you have a sensitive skin and are prone to allergies, it is best to test an essential oil before using it. Put one drop of the essential oil in the crook of your elbow. If you experience no reaction within an hour, it is safe to use.
- Citric essential oils are photosensitive. If applying lemon essential oil, do not sit in the sun, or you could develop permanent marks on your skin.
- If you accidentally get essential oil in your eyes, do not rinse with water; use a carrier oil instead, which your tears will then dilute.
- Never leave bottles of essential oil within reach of children.

CAUTION
Industry guidelines regarding the ingestion of essential oils vary from country to country. We therefore recommend you consult an appropriately qualified aromatherapist before using any remedies marked with an asterisk.*

TAKE NOTE
TERMS USED

Essential oil   concentrated, volatile plant oil

Carrier oil   the oil with which an essential oil is diluted

Infused oil   a carrier oil infused with beneficial plant material, such as arnica, calendula, or St John's wort (hypericum); sometimes termed 'macerated' oils.

1 tsp (teaspoon) = 5 ml
1 tbsp (tablespoon) = 15 ml

Essential oils tend to be sold in two types of bottle, with different droppers (pipettes). With the normal, regular size droppers, around 20 drops of essential oil = 1 ml. However, other bottles have fine or thin-tipped droppers that produce around 40 drops per ml. When you buy essential oils, make sure that you know precisely what size dropper they come with.

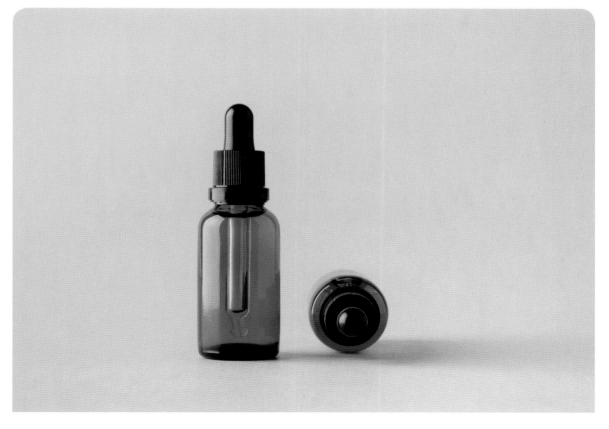

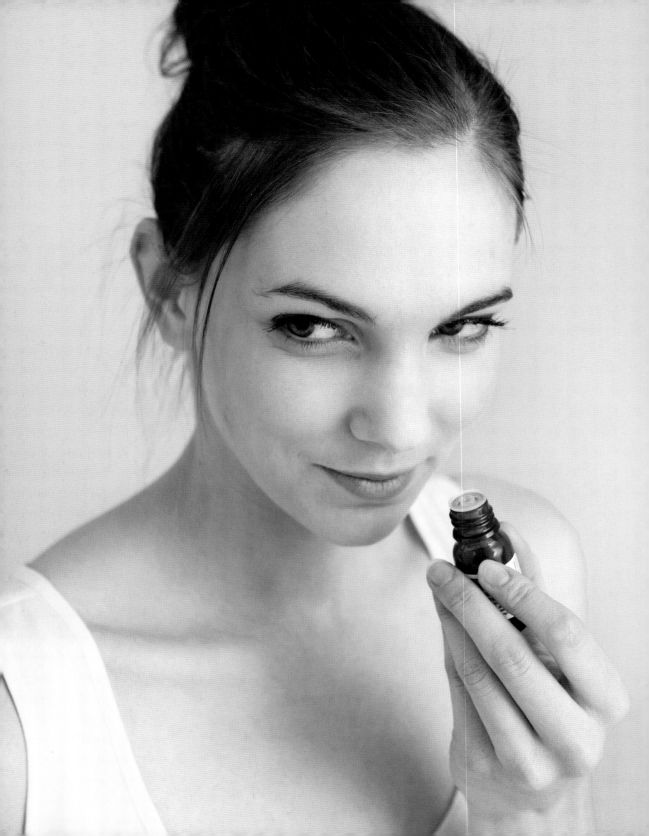

PART 1

YOUR 6 INDISPENSABLE ESSENTIAL OILS

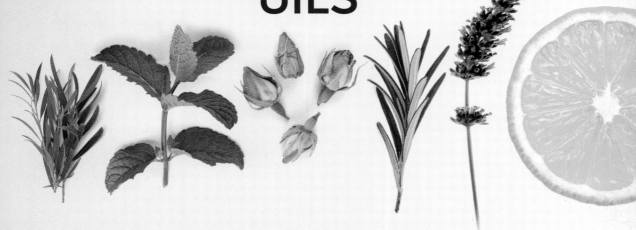

Here, unveiled, are the top six essential oils. First is tea tree, which has outstanding healing powers. Next comes lemon, a purifying force in beauty care, well-being, and the home. Then, there's lovely lavender, with its enchanting fragrance, and peppermint, a first-aid star. Rosemary cineole is effective for respiratory conditions and skin care, and, lastly, damask rose brings a beautifying touch and calms a troubled mind.

TEA TREE

THE MULTI-PURPOSE HOME REMEDY

Tea tree, despite its name, has nothing to do with tea. It is native to Australia where the Aboriginal people have traditionally used it as a strong antimicrobial remedy to combat infections. That power to protect and cure makes it one of our chosen essential oils. It should be part of every first aid kit as each drop has such a strong antiseptic effect.

Whether it's a cut that won't heal, lingering sinusitis, or a general infection, there is so much that tea tree oil can treat. You should also keep it in the bathroom – and not just for its fresh, green fragrance of camphor. It also has a soothing, purifying, cleansing effect on the skin: it treats all sorts of skin disorders including acne, bites, burns, and fungal infections. It can be added to baths, showers, and soaps, enhancing them with its fresh aroma and natural antibacterial properties, and is equally effective in the laundry room; here, combined with a natural household soap, it will refresh your clothes and bed linen. You can even use it to clean pets' toys. When used in a spray or diffuser, it will work its cleansing magic throughout the house; it will kill off bugs that attack your plants, too. Everyone can benefit from the disinfecting and antiseptic power of this essential oil.

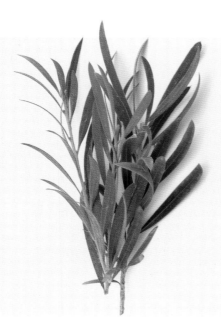

PROFILE

Botanical name *Melaleuca alternifolia*

Family Myrtaceae

Origin Australia, South Africa

Plant part used Leaves

Aroma Camphorated, fresh

Flavour Astringent, slightly bitter, and spicy

Principal biochemical constituents
Monoterpenoids: terpinen-4-ol
Monoterpenes

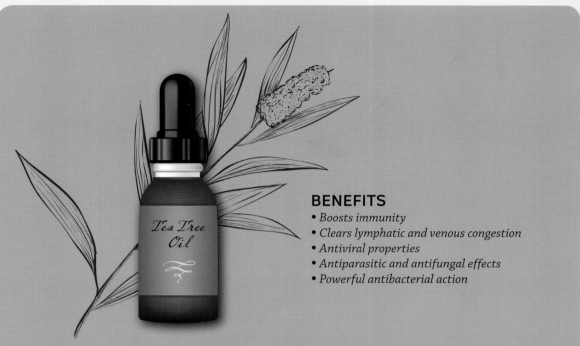

BENEFITS
- *Boosts immunity*
- *Clears lymphatic and venous congestion*
- *Antiviral properties*
- *Antiparasitic and antifungal effects*
- *Powerful antibacterial action*

APPLICATIONS

BEAUTY CARE
- It clears, cleanses, and purifies the skin.

FOR MIND AND BODY
- It combats respiratory infections, such as flu, fever, colds, rhinitis, bronchitis, and sinusitis. It also strengthens the immune system.
- It acts as an expectorant, helping to loosen mucus.
- Its antiseptic effect prevents wound infections.
- It soothes the pain of insect bites, burns, and sunburn.
- It is effective against skin, digestive, and vaginal fungal infections.
- It treats cystitis.

IN YOUR HOME
- It purifies the air you breathe.
- It kills germs on linen and bedclothes.
- It lets you clean the natural way, without using synthetic products.

CAUTION Tea tree oil is well tolerated and can be used diluted on the skin, diffused into the air, and, in an appropriate solution, can be ingested, too*.

LEMON

THE GREAT PURIFIER

Lemon essential oil is easily added to beneficial beauty creams, giving it the chance to work its magic, toning your skin and combating fluid retention. It operates at a deep level, strengthening blood vessel walls and making them more flexible. It also combats rosacea (red, hypersensitive skin). Its antiseptic and air-purifying properties are valuable for fighting off respiratory infections, especially in winter.

The essential oil can also work wonders for an immune system under strain and for those whose feet and hands are ultrasensitive to the cold. If you take a close look at its various applications, it is easy to see why it is such a favourite with many women. It combats acne, treats greasy skin, brightens the dullest complexion, corrects greasy hair, helps smooth away wrinkles, tones and whitens nails, and gets rid of accumulated fat – and that's just beauty care! Lemon essential oil is as highly valued for its household magic. Its ultra-powerful grease-removing, whitening, and descaling properties easily rival those of commercial cleaning products, but it works without damaging the planet – simply adding the fresh, citrus fragrance of its sun-ripened fruit. Tough in the war against microbes and bacteria, and pitiless when repelling mites and ants, lemon essential oil can be used everywhere in the home.

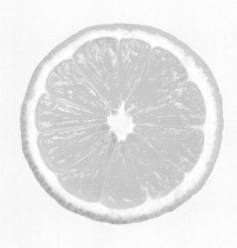

PROFILE

Botanical name *Citrus limon, Citrus limonum*

Family Rutaceae

Origin Mediterranean Basin

Plant part used Zest (from the rind of the fruit)

Aroma Fresh, vibrant, sweet, mild

Flavour Acidic and slightly bitter

Principal biochemical constituents
Monoterpenes: limonene

BENEFITS

- *Boosts the immune system*
- *General antimicrobial action*
- *Improves digestion*
- *Calms the nervous system*

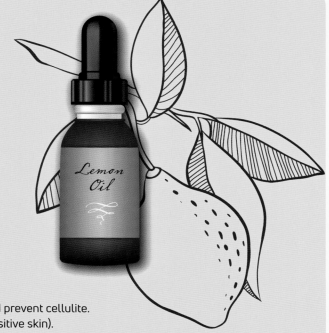

APPLICATIONS

BEAUTY CARE

- It helps to eliminate excess fat and prevent cellulite.
- It combats rosacea (red, hypersensitive skin).
- It treats acne and corrects greasy skin.
- It brightens the complexion and smooths out wrinkles.
- It is especially useful for hand and nail care.

FOR MIND AND BODY

- It cleanses the liver and the digestive system
- It treats respiratory infections, such as colds, flu, sinusitis, and bronchitis, and limits their duration.
- It calms and reduces morning sickness.
- It boosts blood circulation.
- It combats general fatigue and loss of concentration.

IN YOUR HOME

- It has an antiseptic effect and purifies the air.
- It gets rid of mites and ants.

CAUTION Essential oils derived from citrus fruits (sometimes called 'essences' because they are obtained by cold-pressing the rind to extract the zest rather than by distillation) are highly phototoxic. This means that they sensitize the skin to the sun's rays, which can cause unsightly pigmentation. Whether it's lemon, mandarin, grapefruit, orange, or bergamot, do not use a citrus-based essential oil in the 12 hours before you sunbathe. They are rich in chemicals called terpenes and can burn the skin if they are not sufficiently diluted.

LAVENDER

THE SUPREME ESSENTIAL OIL

Its name alone evokes fields of glorious purple in the French region of Provence between Drôme, Mount Ventoux, Luberon, and the canyon of Verdon. Here, to the sound of cicadas, lavender exudes the fragrance so highly prized by the great perfumers. The familiar aroma is also widely used – perhaps overused – by industrial manufacturers but often in a synthetic form which does nothing for health or well-being.

The true essential oil of lavender is something quite different – almost a cure-all, given the many different conditions it can treat. From head to toe, it heals, pampers, destroys germs, relaxes, tones, and purifies. It is the most versatile of all essential oils, the one which relieves a multitude of problems. It has another asset, too. Unlike other essential oils, it can be applied directly to the skin without being mixed with a carrier oil. It's also safe to use (in various forms) with pets, too. As a further bonus, this supreme essential oil can also help you look after your home. Its antibacterial action makes it a miracle product for bathrooms and toilets, and when mixed with vinegar, it creates a delightfully scented fabric conditioner for your laundry.

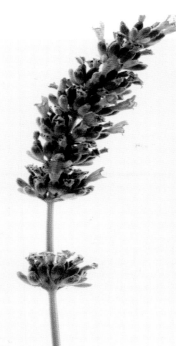

PROFILE

Botanical name *Lavandula angustifolia, Lavandula officinalis, Lavandula vera*

Family Lamiaceae

Origin South of France

Plant part used Flower spikes

Aroma Fresh, flowery, with a sweet hint of camphor, slightly minty

Flavour Spicy, hot, and slightly bitter

Principal biochemical constituents
Monoterpenoids: linalol
Esters: linalyl acetate

BENEFITS
- *Regulates the nervous system*
- *Antispasmodic, relaxing*
- *Soothes, calms, antidepressant*
- *Antiseptic and wound-healing*

APPLICATIONS

BEAUTY CARE
- It soothes skin irritation and a dry, itchy scalp.
- It tones and softens skin.
- It treats acne.
- It is suitable for all skin types – it restores the skin's balance.
- It is especially good for treating sensitive skin.

FOR MIND AND BODY
- It has an anti-inflammatory and analgesic effect, helping to relieve disorders such as migraine, toothache, and stomach pain.
- It has antimicrobial and wound-healing properties, treating wounds and problems such as skin ulcers, burns, irritated skin, itchiness, and infectious or allergic dermatitis.
- It relaxes muscles, helping to relieve conditions such as cramp or contractures.
- It alleviates the stinging pain and irritation of insect and animal bites.

IN YOUR HOME
- Its lovely, 'clean' fragrance can be used to freshen your laundry, cupboards, vacuum cleaner, shoes, and every room in the house.
- You can use its scent on writing paper. Like all essential oils, it isn't greasy and doesn't stain. Try pouring a few drops of essential oil onto a piece of fabric or paper. The next day there will be no visible trace.

CAUTION Gentle, non-toxic lavender is a friend to all the family. Young children and even babies tolerate it perfectly. It can be used directly on the skin, in a spray, or ingested*. However, don't forget the crook-of-the-elbow test (see page 8), as some people may be allergic to the essential oil.

PEPPERMINT

THE PAIN RELIEVER

Migraine, painful periods, a blow, bump, or other injury – peppermint essential oil is the best fragrant treatment for pain. It's a first-aid star, a first response treatment that soothes the pain of knocks and reduces bruising. It is equally valued for its ability to settle digestive problems.

Whether it's food poisoning, nausea, dizziness, or liver congestion, peppermint essential oil will help cleanse the digestive system, treat disorders, and also ensure that your breath is fresh. Together with lemon essential oil, it has a further talent that is greatly appreciated in an era of junk food and pollution of every kind: it detoxifies the body. On the beauty-care front, peppermint essential oil can also be used in many ways – as part of a 'wake-up' shower gel, or a cold, refreshing, invigorating rub, or in a massage oil to revive tired feet. Like all essential oils, peppermint has antibacterial properties, which make it effective against winter respiratory disorders and equally useful as a refreshing deodorant. When diffused in a room, it also cleanses the air.

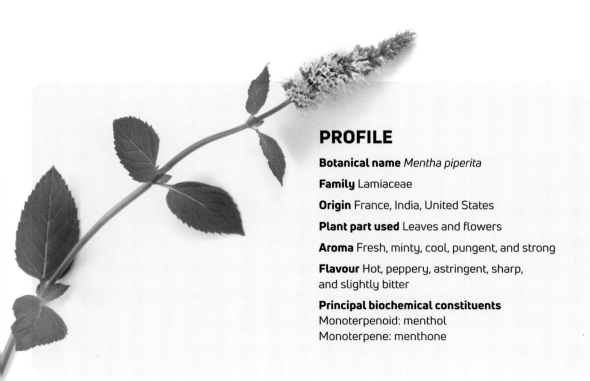

PROFILE

Botanical name *Mentha piperita*

Family Lamiaceae

Origin France, India, United States

Plant part used Leaves and flowers

Aroma Fresh, minty, cool, pungent, and strong

Flavour Hot, peppery, astringent, sharp, and slightly bitter

Principal biochemical constituents
Monoterpenoid: menthol
Monoterpene: menthone

BENEFITS

- *General, cardiac and digestive*
- *Anaesthetic and analgesic stimulant*
- *Eases liver congestion*
- *Refreshes*

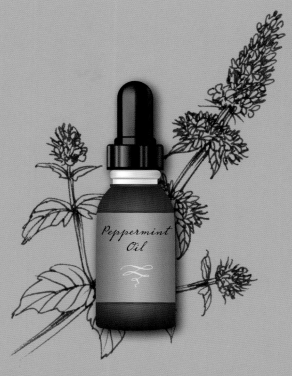

APPLICATIONS

BEAUTY CARE

- It adds a delightful, cooling touch to cosmetic treatments.
- It combats excessive perspiration.

FOR MIND AND BODY

- It has a strong anaesthetic effect, relieving period pains, migraines, and the soreness of injuries.
- It treats digestive disorders and keeps breath fresh.
- It has antimicrobial and antibacterial properties.
- It prevents nausea and travel sickness.
- It soothes headaches and calms stress.

IN YOUR HOME

- It gets rid of mosquitoes, flies, and mites.

CAUTION You must not use it neat on a large area of skin; it has too great a cooling effect and could produce hypothermia. For widespread use, it must be diluted with other essential oils and an appropriate amount of carrier oil before application.

Mothers-to-be should not use it at all during pregnancy, nor until after they have finished breastfeeding. Peppermint essential oil is poisonous for babies and infants. It should not be given to children under seven years old, especially by mouth.

People who are receiving homeopathic care should wait at least two hours after a treatment before using peppermint essential oil. When ingested, it can reduce the effects of homeopathy.

ROSEMARY CINEOLE

THE ENT EXPERT

Food-lovers are familiar with rosemary because of its role in a bouquet garni; together with thyme, laurel, savory, and other regional herbs, it adds a distinctive flavour to a variety of dishes including casseroles and stews.

On the medical front, ear, nose, and throat (ENT) disorders – sore throats, earache, rhinitis, flu, colds, or phlegmy coughs – are its speciality; it can treat them all effectively. Rosemary essential oil has beauty-care attributes, too. It cleans and conditions hair, and also helps invigorate older or tired skin, or young problem skin, thanks to its stimulating, firming, and healing properties. Its astringent power and ability to restore radiance and elasticity can benefit everyone. In the garden, rosemary and its essential oil help to protect plants and flowers from aphid attacks.

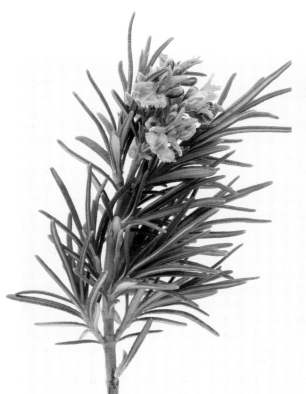

PROFILE

Botanical name *Rosmarinus officinalis*

Family Lamiaceae

Origin Corsica

Plant part used Flowering sprigs

Aroma Fresh, herbaceous, camphorated with a hint of pine and deep woody notes

Flavour Sharp, bittersweet, and lightly astringent

Principal biochemical constituents
Terpenoid oxide: 1,8-cineole
Monoterpene: alpha-pinene
Monoterpenol: borneol

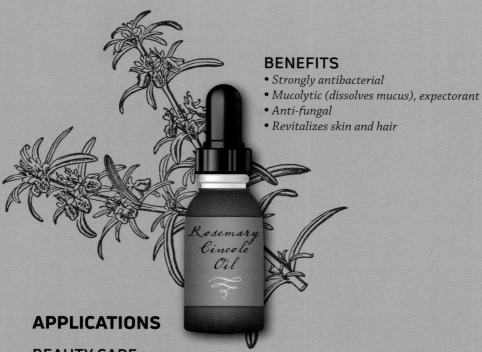

BENEFITS
- *Strongly antibacterial*
- *Mucolytic (dissolves mucus), expectorant*
- *Anti-fungal*
- *Revitalizes skin and hair*

APPLICATIONS

BEAUTY CARE
- It tones the scalp and boosts hair growth.
- It has a stimulating and firming action on mature skin.
- It speeds healing.
- It has astringent properties, helping skin regain its elasticity.

FOR MIND AND BODY
- It combats all ENT (ear, nose, and throat) infections.
- It effectively treats cystitis and thrush.
- It helps counter chronic fatigue, abnormal physical weakness or lack of energy, and physical or mental burnout.

IN YOUR HOME
- It freshens and disinfects every room.
- In the laundry, it adds its fragrance to clothes and other items.
- It protects plants from aphids.

CAUTION Usually safe, but consult a qualified aromatherapist before using if pregnant, or if you have epilepsy or high blood pressure.

DAMASK ROSE

THE PRECIOUS ONE

With its sophisticated, sweet, velvety fragrance, damask rose essential oil is not one to waste on household chores. It is just as well that it does not have any great ability to disinfect the home or remove limescale, as it costs about 30 times more than other essential oils!

What makes damask rose so special and so worthy of inclusion in our selection is its talent for revitalizing dry, sensitive, or greasy skin by stimulating the production of new cells. There is also its anti-wrinkle action and its ability to give a complexion an instant boost of radiance and a rosy touch of colour, with skin so smooth it seems ironed. In addition to its capacity for pampering and looking after our appearance, it is also notable for relieving insomnia, calming anxiety, defusing anger, and alleviating sorrow. Damask rose essential oil can keep us balanced, calming stress and boosting our general sense of well-being. It also encourages our libido, combating impotence and low sex drive with its aphrodisiac powers. In a general way, it also supports our sense of worth, protecting against depression and lack of confidence. This essential oil may not be the best household aid, but when added to the water in a steam-iron or diffused in a baby's bedroom, it creates a peaceful atmosphere with a delicious fragrance of rose petals.

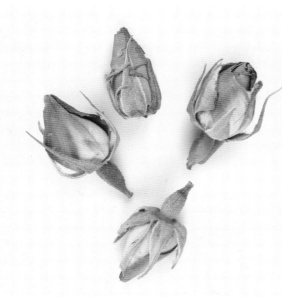

PROFILE

Botanical name *Rosa damascena*

Family Rosaceae

Origin Bulgaria, Morocco, Turkey

Plant part used Petals

Aroma Subtle and flowery

Flavour Sweet, like honey

Principal biochemical constituents
Monoterpenoid: citronellol, geraniol, nerol

BENEFITS

- *Astringent, tones and invigorates skin*
- *Prevents wrinkles*
- *Combats depression, insomnia, and anxiety*
- *Powerfully fragrant*

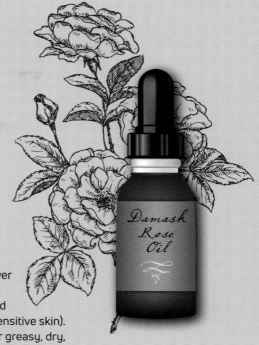

APPLICATIONS

BEAUTY CARE

- It has an anti-ageing effect; its regenerating power stimulates the production of new skin cells.
- It is astringent, an excellent tonic for the skin, and a treatment to consider for rosacea (red, hypersensitive skin).
- It can work marvels on any type of skin; whether greasy, dry, or mature, it can soothe, repair, soften, revitalize, and more.
- Its rich fragrance envelops the skin like a luxurious, delicate veil.

FOR MIND AND BODY

- It treats psychological issues that stem from gynaecological and hormonal problems.
- It prevents postnatal depression and helps sufferers fight back
- It combats eczema
- It effectively relieves insomnia, anxiety, grief, anger, and other troubling emotions.

IN YOUR HOME

- A few drops added to the water in a steam-iron impart a delicate fragrance to clothes and linen.
- Two drops on a child's pillow will encourage peaceful sleep.

CAUTION As mentioned earlier, essential oils must be kept out of reach of children. Be especially careful with damask rose, as children will be attracted by its sweet perfume. (To avoid giving you a shock, this is an idea of its price: around £30–50 /US$40–65 for just 5 ml – and it can cost even more. But it will bring you pleasure for months, even years.)

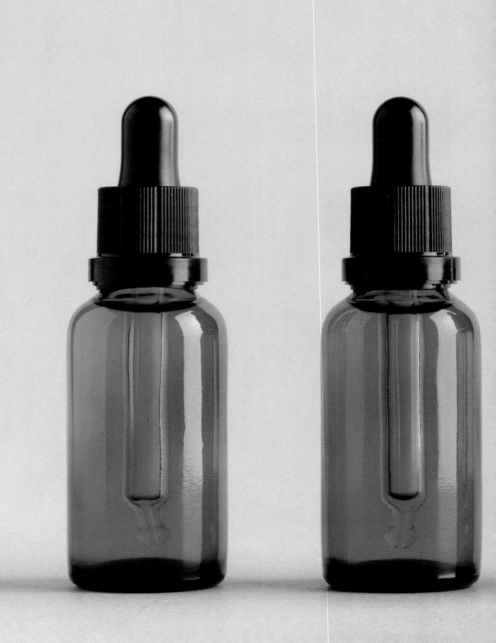

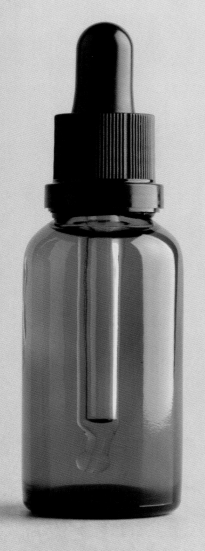

PART 2

HOW TO USE THE OILS

The fun begins. In 'Beauty care', you'll learn how to mix and apply fragrant massage and bath oils, shower gels, body scrubs, and nourishing moisturizers. Essential oils also offer sun protection, as well as hand, foot, face, and hair care, plus tailor-made skin solutions for different age groups. Their healing powers are revealed in 'Looking after mind and body', with precise dosages that must be followed to ensure each remedy is effective and safe. Lastly, it is the turn of your home, garden, and pets to benefit from the unique powers of these six essential oils.

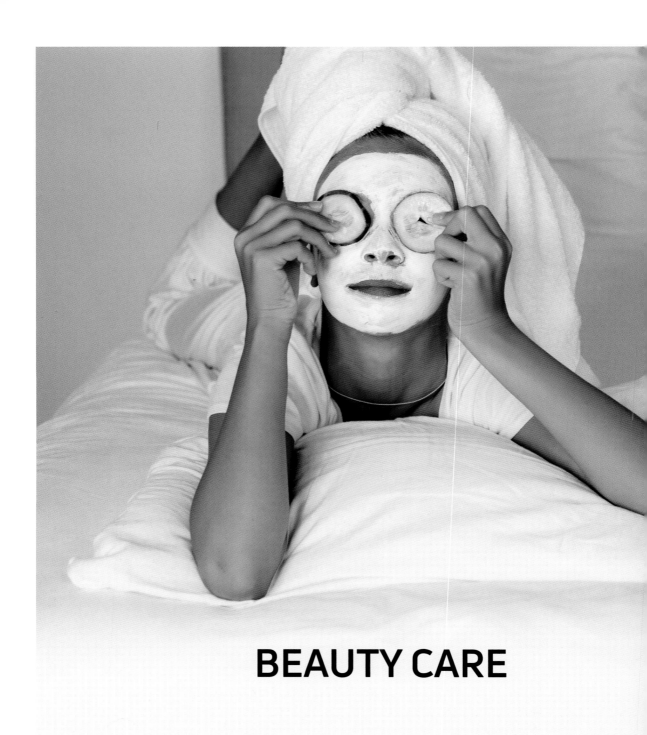

BEAUTY CARE

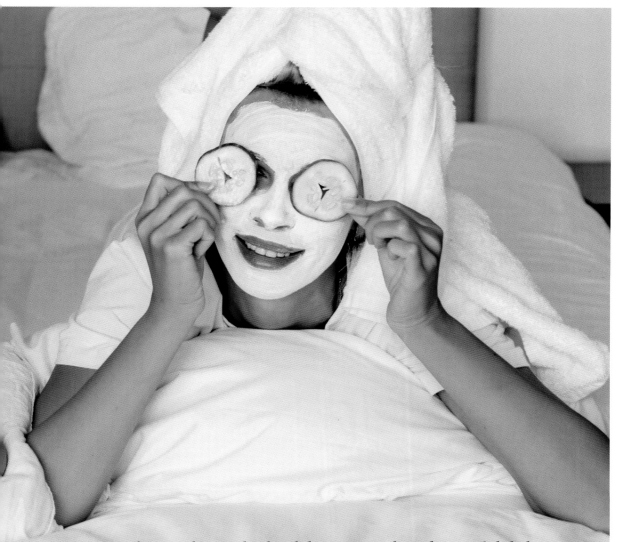

Women have spoken out loud and clear against the inclusion of phthalates, formaldehyde, parabens, and other chemical preservatives widely used in commercial cosmetics. So now is an excellent time to start preparing your own beauty-care products, without spending a fortune, by taking advantage of the natural qualities of essential oils and their detoxifying, strengthening, and toning properties. A few drops of the appropriate essential oil, a suitable carrier oil, no preservatives, and a fragrance that comes straight from nature – it's all there to give you the pleasure of creating an array of cosmetics to suit your tastes and needs.

BODY CARE

FRAGRANT MASSAGES

The application of essential oils to the skin is very popular in aromatherapy and often highly effective. The essential oil is quickly absorbed, but its action is progressive and long-lasting. The active substances work both on the skin and at a deeper level, because they can penetrate skin layers and circulate throughout the body. As a result, it is via the skin that essential oil beauty care and therapeutic treatments are most frequently applied.

Essential oils are, however, powerful; if used in their purest form, they can cause irritation. This is why they are always mixed with a carrier oil before being applied in a massage. Allow 20 drops of essential oil per 2 tsp of carrier oil. Next, comes the decision of which essential oil, or essential oils to choose, as – depending on the effect desired – it is possible to mix two or more essential oils and also to use one or several carrier oils.

THE TOOLS YOU NEED
TO PREPARE A TREATMENT

1 bottle of essential oil (or up to 4 different types)
1 bottle of carrier oil
1 clean, empty 10 ml (⅓ fl oz) bottle, made of dark, coloured glass

TAKE CARE

- **Always wash your hands** thoroughly before and after every fragrant massage – even if it's a quick one. Before the massage, of course, as a hygienic measure, as it would be a shame to contaminate the essential oil/ carrier oil mixture. Why you should do it afterwards is less obvious, but equally worth noting for your safety. If you get distracted, forget that you've been handling essential oils, and suddenly need to scratch an itching eye, you could get a nasty surprise.
- **Skin test**. Is yours the kind of skin that comes out in a rash when you put on the smallest plaster? If so, it is probably sensible to carry out the skin test indicated on page 8, using your chosen essential oil/carrier oil mixture, before you apply it to a larger area.
- **Use high-quality oils** in your preparations. Ensure that your essential oils are 100 per cent natural and that the carrier oils are cold pressed and organic.
- **Never use an essential oil** that has not been adequately diluted on areas of the body covered by a mucous membrane, such as the nostrils, inside of the mouth, the vagina, and anus, unless advised to do so by a qualified aromatherapist (as occasionally with tea tree and lavender essential oils).
- **Don't jump in the shower** straight after a fragrant massage. Wrap yourself in a cosy, warm bathrobe for at least 10 minutes to let the essential oil do its work. Then carry on with whatever you have to do, or slip under your bedcovers, depending on the time of day.
- **A massage should always** be applied in the same direction as blood circulates back to the heart.

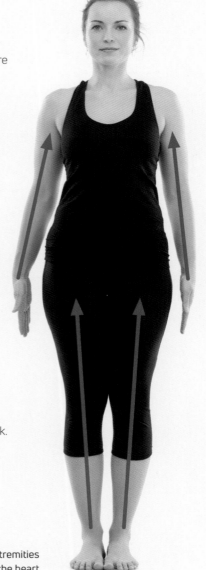

Massage from the extremities
towards the heart

CARRIER OILS

Essential oils blend easily with carrier oils, losing none of their attributes. Any carrier oil can be used to dilute an essential oil, but one clever choice is to select a carrier oil whose properties also enhance beauty, well-being, or general health. Look at their profiles to understand what they can do.

SWEET ALMOND Softening power

A perfect, light oil for dry, sensitive skins, sweet almond has a subtle, light fragrance. It is great for delicate skin, such as children's, and hydrates and nourishes. It is equally suitable for irritated, problem skin, and even eczema-prone skin and stretch marks, as it soothes and restores firmness.

ARGAN Rejuvenating from head to toe

In Morocco, women have long known of its incomparable benefits and passed its secrets down from generation to generation. In the West, too, over the past few years, it has become highly prized for its beneficial effects. It's a self-contained beauty kit – combating ageing skin, wrinkles, hair loss, and more. Its revitalizing power can fight off all the ravages of time. It repairs, strengthens, and stimulates the production of hydrophobic lipid components in the hydrolipidic film that protects the skin, reinforcing its natural barrier effect. Get to know it before choosing it for your massage; some people don't like its aroma.

TAMANU Boosting blood and lymph flow

Also known as calophyllum oil (as it comes from the fruit kernel of the Southeast Asian tamanu tree, *Calophyllum inophyllum*), tamanu oil encourages good circulation. It helps relieve varicose veins, haemorrhoids, rosacea (red, hypersensitive skin), and all other circulatory disorders. It is useful in massage treatments for swollen, aching legs – peripheral arterial disease, in which the build-up of fatty deposits in the arteries restricts blood supply to leg muscles. More generally, it has a draining effect, boosting the flow of blood and lymph around the body. Its antimicrobial properties can also work wonders on problem or damaged skin. Its aroma is a mixture of nuts and curry, and it has a quite singular consistency, tending to solidify at temperatures below 25°C (77°F), although this does not affect its quality. If it does go solid, simply stand the bottle in some warm water. It is best to warm it before application to aid absorption.

MACADAMIA Perfect for massages

It has a gentle fragrance, with a nutty hint, and two drops in the crook of your arm are quickly absorbed into the skin. That's an especially valuable attribute; who wants to come away from a massage with their body covered in an oily film? With macadamia oil, there's no risk of staining your clothes, it is absorbed so rapidly that it leaves the skin quite dry. Its specialist area is the circulation of lymph, so in cases of fluid retention it is useful for tracking down and eliminating cellulite. The oil also helps treat problems such as tired, aching legs, visible little blood vessels, stretch marks, or scars, by boosting circulation, and relaxing and nourishing your skin. One last talent which will please sun-worshippers; macadamia oil offers a little protection against UV rays – a good reason for adding it to your cosmetic collection.

EVENING PRIMROSE AND BORAGE Anti-ageing

This powerful duo will be very familiar to those with more mature skin. The two revitalize the complexion, making skin firmer and brighter. Even better, they encourage hormonal balance and boost cell renewal, a valuable anti-ageing benefit. Both evening primrose and borage are delicate oils; it is best to keep them away from sunlight, which can cause them to deteriorate.

MUSK ROSE OIL FROM CHILE Anti-wrinkle, healing, repairing

Omega 3, omega 6, antioxidants – all constituents of this oil – are a strong indication of its anti-ageing benefits. That is its major role; it has a powerful anti-wrinkle effect. It smooths out older lines and makes newer ones completely disappear. Mixed with rose essential oil, it creates one of the most nourishing and repairing night creams. Used in a massage, it is a balm for the skin. It treats scarring from acne, burns, or an operation, and also stretch marks, sun spots, and age spots, softening, reducing blemishes, and toning tired skin.

SESAME A useful massage aid

This oil is rapidly absorbed by the skin, leaving a silky film that doesn't stain. Its characteristic aroma of roasted seeds is also gentle and pleasant. Its ability to revitalize and soothe irritated skin, and to soften and plump up damaged skin is also significant.

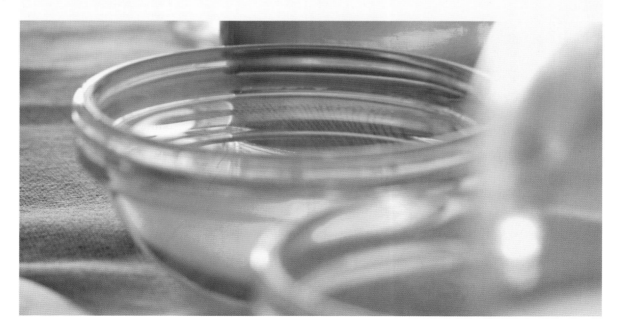

3 GREAT SELF-MASSAGES

Relaxation, comfort, unwinding – that's the promise of a pampering self-massage, a sure way to relieve the stress of a hectic life. As it is absorbed through the skin, the essential oil also releases its molecules, boosting the power of the massage. Massaging the feet, hands, and face is especially soothing.

METHOD
You should generally allow around 20 drops of essential oil per 2 tsp of carrier oil. The mixture is usually made with one or several carrier oils and one or more essential oils. If you prefer a more creamy, less liquid consistency, go for a massage balm. Melt some shea butter, bain-marie style, by putting the butter in a bowl, then placing the bowl in a saucepan containing about 4 cm (just over 1 in) of simmering water, whisking constantly. When it is smooth, take it off the heat and mix in the essential oil or oils, stirring until the solution is thick and creamy.

A FIRMING FACIAL MASSAGE
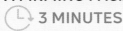 3 MINUTES

Add 5 drops **lavender essential oil**, 3 drops **damask rose essential oil**, and 2 drops **lemon essential oil** to 1 tsp musk rose carrier oil, and mix well.

- Pour a little of this solution into your hand, then spread it over the whole of your face and neck, avoiding your eyelids.
- Place both hands on your chin and, keeping the palms flat, lightly massage the skin, slowly moving upwards towards the cheeks.
- Next, place your hands in the centre of your forehead and massage outwards towards your temples.
- Using your thumbs, smooth along your eyebrows, moving from the centre towards the edge of your face.
- Gently pat your cheeks, working from your nose out to your ears. Lightly squeezing the skin between your thumb and forefinger, work along the jawbone, from the ears to the centre of the chin.
- Do this massage only at night, as the lemon essential oil can increase the skin's sensitivity to the sun.

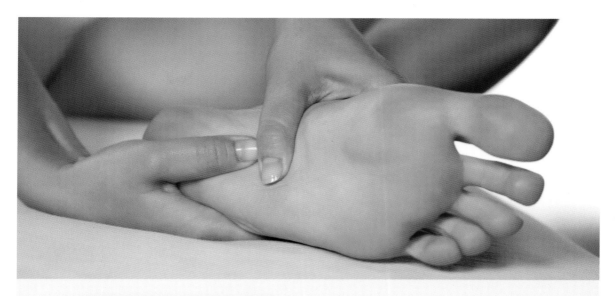

SOOTHING FOOT MASSAGE

 5 MINUTES

Mix 1 tsp hazelnut carrier oil with 10 drops **lavender essential oil**.

- Sitting comfortably, raise one foot and rest it on the opposite thigh.
- Pour a little of the mixture into one hand, then take hold of the raised foot with both hands. Smooth the oils over the foot, starting from the toes and working towards the ankle.
- Using circular movements, press your thumb along the sole of the foot and over the heel.
- Close your hand and roll your fist firmly along the underside of your foot, still working from the toes towards the heel.
- Finally, take your foot in both hands and apply pressure to the whole area, from the toes to the heel. Change feet and repeat.

PAMPERING HAND MASSAGE

4 MINUTES

Mix 10 drops **lemon essential oil** and 1 tsp macadamia carrier oil.

- Pour a little of the preparation into the palm of your hand, then warm it by rubbing your hands together.
- Using the thumb of one hand, massage the palm of the other, pressing down firmly and working from the centre outwards.
- Now, take your wrist and massage the back of the hand, working towards the fingertips.
- Finish by massaging each finger, one after the other, from the fingertips down to the wrist.
- Use this massage only at night, as lemon essential oil can increase the skin's sensitivity to the sun.

3 GREAT SLIMMING MASSAGES

The goal is to reshape your body's contours. How can essential oils help you do that? By toning, firming, and strengthening the skin, and flushing out the system to help get rid of waste products and break down fatty tissue. The combination of massage and essential oils is perfect for this. By stimulating blood and lymph circulation, an essential oil massage speeds up the elimination process, helping to remove stored fat, water, and cellulite.

Use about 20 drops essential oil to 2 tsp of carrier oil.

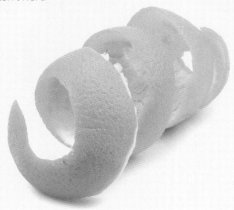

FIRM BUTTOCKS
4 MINUTES

Mix 10 drops **rosemary cineole essential oil** and 5 drops **lemon essential oil** with 1 tsp Isopropyl (rubbing) alcohol 70% and 1 tsp macadamia carrier oil. Shake well before application.

- Pour a little of the mixture into the palm of your hand, and warm it by rubbing one hand against the other.
- Grasp a fold of flesh at the top of your thigh, and press and roll it upwards towards the top of your buttock.
- Repeat three times on each buttock.
- Then take a buttock in each hand and knead firmly. You should definitely be able to feel the heat, but it shouldn't hurt.

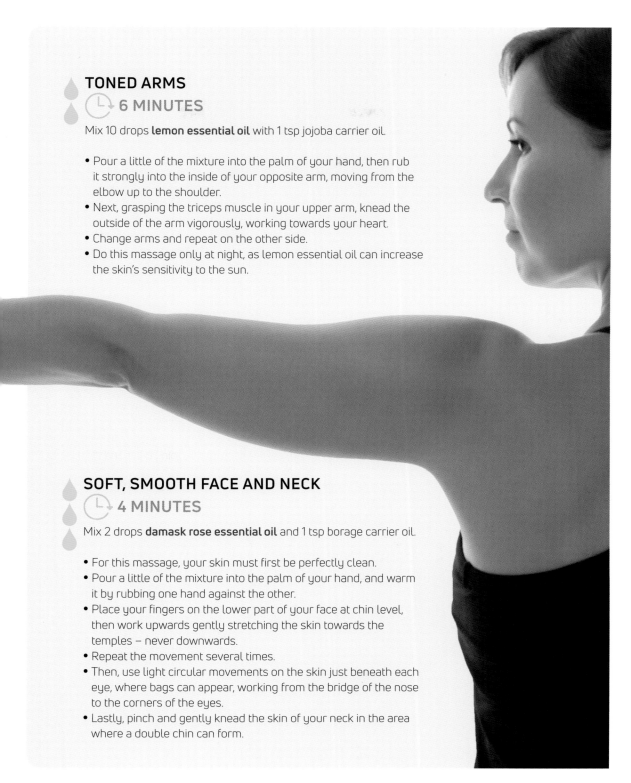

TONED ARMS
⏱ 6 MINUTES

Mix 10 drops **lemon essential oil** with 1 tsp jojoba carrier oil.

- Pour a little of the mixture into the palm of your hand, then rub it strongly into the inside of your opposite arm, moving from the elbow up to the shoulder.
- Next, grasping the triceps muscle in your upper arm, knead the outside of the arm vigorously, working towards your heart.
- Change arms and repeat on the other side.
- Do this massage only at night, as lemon essential oil can increase the skin's sensitivity to the sun.

SOFT, SMOOTH FACE AND NECK
⏱ 4 MINUTES

Mix 2 drops **damask rose essential oil** and 1 tsp borage carrier oil.

- For this massage, your skin must first be perfectly clean.
- Pour a little of the mixture into the palm of your hand, and warm it by rubbing one hand against the other.
- Place your fingers on the lower part of your face at chin level, then work upwards gently stretching the skin towards the temples – never downwards.
- Repeat the movement several times.
- Then, use light circular movements on the skin just beneath each eye, where bags can appear, working from the bridge of the nose to the corners of the eyes.
- Lastly, pinch and gently knead the skin of your neck in the area where a double chin can form.

FRAGRANT BATHS

Which beauty treatment can treat and take care of you while providing the most delightful relaxation? A bath scented with fragrant essential oils. Buoyed by the water, our bodies feel light, joints relax, muscles unwind, pores open, and our minds feel free. This is also the moment when essential oils can employ their most effective constituents. Depending on which essential oil you choose, you can give yourself a detox, fat-burning, or exfoliating bath – all the while enjoying the delightful fragrances.

WHAT YOU WILL NEED

Essential oils are not water-soluble. Poured neat into water, they will burn your skin. First you have to mix them with a substance that disperses in the bath and combines with the essential oil. You can buy either a bath oil base or you can use a natural emulsifier such as sea salt, bicarbonate of soda, Epsom salts, or Dead Sea salt.

BATH OIL BASE

This can be found in pharmacies, health stores, or online. Use 1 tbsp base oil to 10 drops essential oil. This is by far the best dispersant for essential oils.

SEA SALT

With its cleansing, mineral-rich properties, sea salt works well with essential oils. Pour 10 drops of essential oil onto a handful of salt, then add to bathwater.

BICARBONATE OF SODA

This is used in a similar way to sea salt and, as a bonus, it has a softening and antifungal action. Pour 10 drops of essential oil onto a handful of bicarbonate of soda and add to bathwater.

To soothe aching legs or tired feet, pour 5 drops of essential oil over 3 tbsp bicarbonate, then add to a bowl or footbath of warm water.

EPSOM SALTS AND DEAD SEA SALT

The relaxing, calming, healing action of these two salts will combine with the benefits of the essential oils. Pour 10 drops of essential oil onto a handful of Epsom or Dead Sea salts, then add to bathwater.

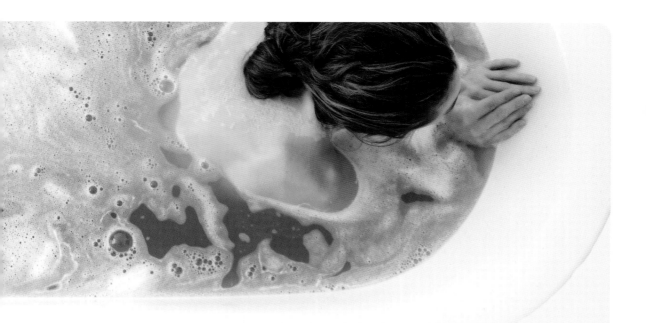

METHOD

This will require a little organization, but just consider the rewards – the pleasure of thinking about nothing, of letting your mind wander in the swirling steam and fragrance, as your body unwinds, calms, and becomes ever lighter.

- Banish the phone, children, and the dog, and announce loud and clear that no one can disturb you, 'I MEAN NO ONE!' for the next hour.
- Keep the implements you need close to hand, such as a bath brush, body scrubber, and exfoliator.
- Make yourself a relaxing herbal tea, then shut yourself off in the bathroom.
- Mix your essential oils with whichever base you choose (see opposite), run the water to a maximum temperature of 38°C (100.4°F), then pour in the mixture when the bath is ready. Stir the water with your hand.
- Wash your face, then prepare two compresses with the herbal tea to apply to your eyes when you're in the bath.
- Background music is helpful (for example, Mozart works perfectly).
- Immerse yourself in the bath, close your eyes, apply the compresses, and let a feeling of well-being waft over you.
- Wait at least 10 minutes before you start on your beauty treatments, whether you plan to use a scrub, exfoliator, or anything else. Take advantage of this free time and appreciate a moment away from everyday stress.
- After 20 minutes, you should get out of the bath.
- Slip into a bathrobe.

BRILLIANT BATH TREATMENTS

EXFOLIANT

In a bowl, mix together 200 ml (6¾ fl oz) sea salt, 200 ml (6¾ fl oz) bicarbonate of soda, 200 ml (6¾ fl oz) Epsom salts, and 15 drops **lavender essential oil**.

- Run your bathwater (at a temperature of 38°C/100.4°F), pour in the mixture, and relax in the bath for 20 minutes.
- Finish with a warm shower to rinse the salt residue from your skin.

REJUVENATING

Mix 5 drops **lemon essential oil**, 5 drops **lavender essential oil**, and 5 drops **tea tree essential oil** with 1 tbsp bath oil base.

- Pour this into a warm bath (35°C/95°F), then stir it around with your hand.
- Use this only at night, as lemon essential oil can increase the skin's sensitivity to the sun.

SPARKLING

What a day! You come home stressed out and exhausted. You probably have your own strategies for throwing off a bad mood and not letting it contaminate the home atmosphere. Here's another one that is certainly worth trying: a reviving, energizing bath that will dissolve your worries in its light bubbles.

- In a bowl, mix together 2 tbsp bicarbonate of soda and 2 tsp citric acid (available from pharmacies or the Internet). Add 15 drops **lemon essential oil** and 10 drops **peppermint essential oil**. Stir until smooth,, then mix in 6 tbsp Epsom salts.
- When you are ready, run your bath, add 2 tbsp of the sparkling mixture, and immediately jump in.
- Store the rest of the bath treatment in a pretty glass jar with a tightly fastened lid, and keep it to hand – ready for any further bad moods.

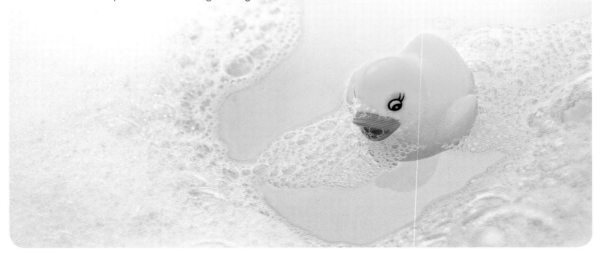

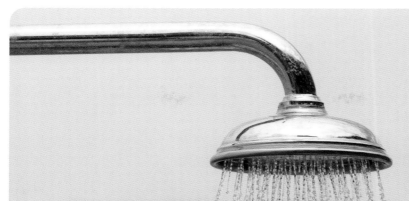

FRAGRANT SHOWERS

Before you go out and brave the world again, do you want to add a spot of pampering to your usual morning routine?

A few drops of essential oil, enveloped in the steam of a hot shower, will give off a perfume that will first awaken your sense of smell and then your whole body. That is the promise of these fragrant treatments. They take no longer than your usual shower, because you can add the essential oils directly to your shower gel. Once you're out of the shower and dry is quite soon enough to start thinking of the thousands of jobs to be done during the day.

METHOD
- Pour a little of your usual shower gel into your hand, add 2 or 3 drops of essential oil, and mix with your finger.
- Apply this to damp skin, massaging it gently, then rinse off.
- Finish by showering yourself with lukewarm water (cold is best but a bit of a shock in the morning) to boost your blood circulation, starting from the feet and working up your body to the shoulders, but concentrating most on the thighs, stomach, and chest.
- Dry yourself gently on your towel, without rubbing.

YOUR OWN PERSONAL SHOWER GEL
You're getting a taste for fragrant showers with essential oils. They've become your morning beauty secret – a moment just for you, as they leave a film of their perfume on your smooth skin. If, at first, you enjoyed experimenting with different essential oils – one day lavender, the next day peppermint – now you know which one (or ones) will work best on your skin. It's time to make a personal shower gel that you can use each morning without having to think about preparing it. Buy a 200 ml (6¾ fl oz) bottle of neutral shower gel base (available at stores that sell natural beauty products, or online), and add 40 drops of essential oil. You can use 40 drops of the same essential oil, or 20 drops each of two different essential oils, or 10 drops each of four different essential oils, but it is best not to mix more than four different essential oils.

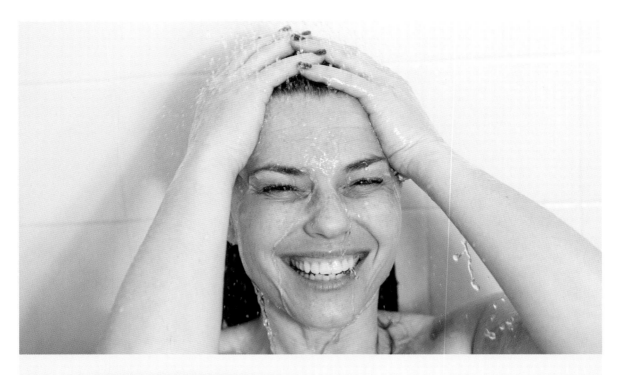

3 GREAT SHOWER GELS

TO SOOTHE TIRED, ACHING LEGS

Mix 2 drops **lemon essential oil** into your usual shower gel and wash yourself, starting with your feet and working up towards your heart. Finish your shower with a blast of lukewarm water (or cold is better!) on your legs: begin with the ankles and work upwards with little circular movements along the thigh to the hip. Then, direct the cold water (which you'll now be used to) onto the sole of one foot and work upwards from the calf to the buttocks for 1 minute, then switch legs. Only take this shower in the evening, as lemon essential oil can increase the skin's sensitivity to the sun.

TO COOL AND REFRESH

This mixture could be your best summer friend. Pour 20 drops **lavender essential oil** and 2 drops **peppermint essential oil** into a clean 250 ml (8½ fl oz) bottle, then top up with neutral shower gel base. Shake well each time before use.

TO WAKE YOU UP

Tough, when it comes to dealing with drowsiness, but gentle on your skin and hair, this shower gel helps you t start the day well. Pour 50 ml (1⅔ fl oz) wheatgerm carrier oil, 20 drops **peppermint essential oil** and 20 drops **lavender essential oil** into a clean 250 ml (8½ fl oz) bottle, and top up with a neutral shower gel base. Shake well each time before use.

FRAGRANT SOAPS

METHOD

- Grate 90 g (3 oz) unscented white Marseille soap (available online or in stores that sell natural beauty products), or use the same weight of soap flakes.
- Melt the soap, using the bain-marie method (see page 32), gently stirring as it warms.
- Mix together the carrier oil and the selected essential oils (choosing whichever inspire you from the preparations below), take the melted soap off the heat, and add your carrier oil/essential oil mixture.
- Stir again. Pour the warm mixture into a silicone mould, and allow it to set and dry for 24 hours before turning it out.

3 GREAT SOAPS

FOR YOUNG SKIN

Mix together 1 tbsp hazelnut carrier oil, 20 drops **tea tree essential oil**, and 20 drops **lemon essential oil**. Stir this into the soap you have melted, once you've taken it off the heat.

FOR DELICATE SKIN

Mix together 1 tbsp sweet almond carrier oil and 40 drops **lavender essential oil**. Stir this into the soap you have melted, once you've taken it off the heat.

FOR EXFOLIATING

Mix together 1 tbsp sweet almond carrier oil, 1 tsp ground almonds, and 20 drops **lemon essential oil**. Stir this into the soap you have melted, once you've taken it off the heat.

HYDROLATES (FLORAL WATERS)

Hydrolates, also known as hydrosols, and floral or herbal waters, should perhaps be called 'essential waters' as, like essential oils, they are made when herbs and flowers are distilled. When the plant matter goes through the still, the process creates two distinct products – the essential oil, which floats on the surface, and, beneath it, the hydrolate (the solution containing water-soluble plant material). Both are full of active constituents from the original plants, though these are much more concentrated in essential oils. Unlike essential oils, floral waters can be used directly on the skin, in a lotion, or as perfume water. They're helpful when creating homemade cosmetics or cooking recipes, because they are much less powerful than essential oils, so can be used more freely, and are light and safe – even for mothers-to-be, breast-feeding mothers, and babies. They can also be ingested.

CHOOSE WISELY

You should not buy anything less than the best. It is eye-opening how often you find impure, diluted, counterfeit, and even contaminated hydrolates. Be firm; buy only products that are 100 per cent organic and preservative free. Just as for essential oils, the scientific species name (for example, *Citrus limonum*, for lemon hydrolate, or lemon floral water) should be mentioned on the label, as well as the specification 'hydrolate', 'hydrosol', 'distillate', or 'distillation' on the label, and note if there are any other added ingredients. If possible, smell the hydrolate; even if its fragrance is not as strong as that of an essential oil, it should be pretty evident. Lastly, price is a good indication: if it is very low, the product is most likely a pale imitation, probably devoid of active constituents, and any health or beauty benefits.

LOOK AFTER THEM PROPERLY

Like essential oils, hydrolates are highly sensitive to sunlight and heat. Because they contain very few aromatic molecules, they also keep less well. Store them in the fridge to avoid variations in temperature and light. Without any preservatives at all, in the cool their active ingredients will remain strong for several months from the date of manufacture; always ask about such details if they don't appear on the bottle label.

WHERE TO BUY THEM

On the high street, the best sources are herbalists, stores that sell organic products, and pharmacies. Online stores are also very useful; some pride themselves on selling products that are 'pure', 'organic', microfiltered, and very reasonably priced. Such sites will also sell everything else required for producing homemade cosmetic products in the best possible way, such as spray bottles, droppers, and bath and shower gel bases. A reputable site will go further with this ecological philosophy, offering hydrolates in recyclable plastic bottles, free of phthalates and bisphenol.

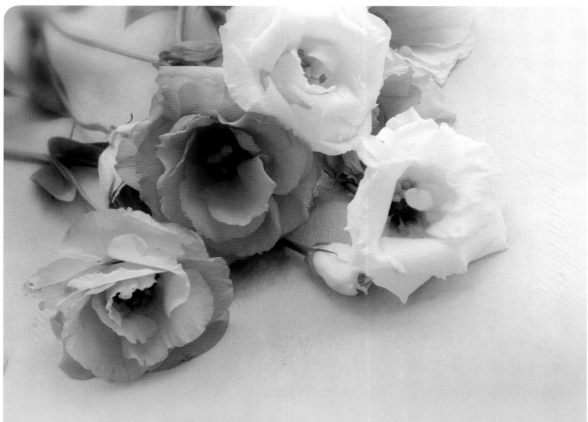

TOP 5 HYDROLATES

- **Lavender** Its calming, clarifying properties soothe irritated skin, sunburn, burns, and more.

- **Rosemary** It refreshes and invigorates both externally (on the skin) and internally (the liver and other internal organs).

- **Rose** Its astringent effect is useful for treating rosacea (red, hypersensitive skin) and eczema.

- **Camomile** It soothes sensitive skin and eye irritation. Taken orally, it prevents worm infections and calms nerves.

- **Orange flower** This hydrolate rejuvenates every skin type. Taken orally, it encourages good sleep.

FRAGRANT EXFOLIANTS

Our poor skin! It's attacked on all sides until it can barely breathe. It tries valiantly to accomplish its huge task of shielding us from environmental enemies, keeping our body temperature stable, and healing wounds, but it works even better when we give it a helping hand.

Moisturizing our skin, oiling it with anti-ageing creams, or putting on makeup are things we do spontaneously because we want to mask the passage of time. But helping the skin to rejuvenate is something we think about less. Essential oils are an excellent way of making exfoliation part of your regular beauty-care regime. Their action is enhanced by the scrub which cleans up the skin by eliminating dead cells and other impurities.

METHOD

The best time to use an exfoliating scrub is before taking a shower or bath, as you have to rinse it off afterwards. Alternatively, it can be applied during a shower: simply wash under the shower, turn it off while applying the scrub, and then rinse. Which raises the question: should you use a scrub on dry or wet skin? It depends on your skin; if it is sensitive, a scrub applied dry can be uncomfortable. Whether using the scrub on dry or wet skin, take a little of the mixture and apply it in circular movements. Concentrate on the hard skin areas, such as knees, elbows and heels. Take your time.

3 GREAT BODY SCRUBS

A REFRESHING SCRUB

Mix 2 tbsp fine table salt, 3 tbsp soft brown sugar, 3 tbsp argan carrier oil, and 3 drops **peppermint essential oil**. Apply to your skin, rub it in, then carefully rinse it off with almost cold water.

AN ANTI-CELLULITE SCRUB

Mix 3 tbsp coffee grounds, 3 tbsp sweet almond carrier oil, and 4 drops **lemon essential oil**. Apply with circular movements to the target areas, such as knees, thighs, buttocks, hips, stomach, or arms. Rinse it off with warm water.

AN ALL-PURPOSE SCRUB

Mix 5 tbsp powdered French green clay and 5 drops **tea tree essential oil** with a little water to make a thick paste. Apply this to damp skin and rub. Rinse well with plenty of warm water, then cold water.

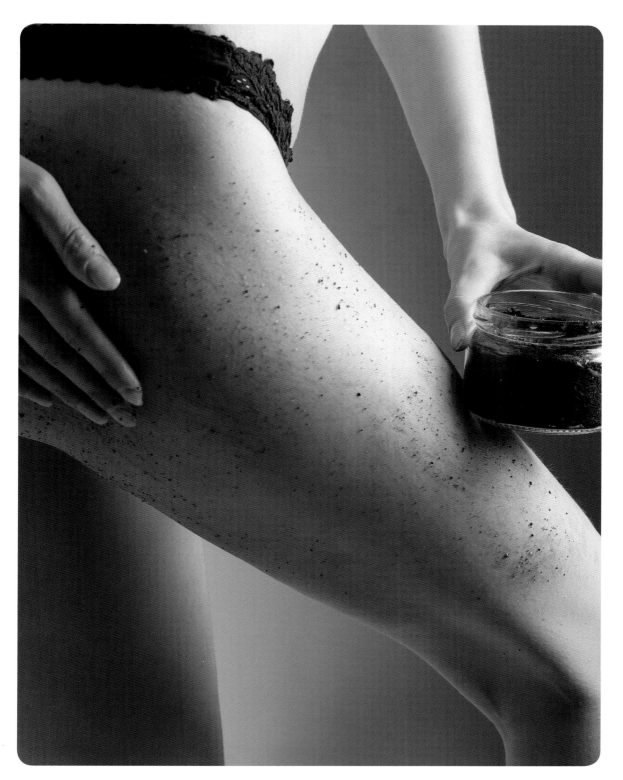

NOURISHING SKIN MOISTURIZERS

If we could have only one beauty product, most of us would choose a moisturizer. A moisturizer is like a second skin.

We put on moisturizer in the morning to protect against the elements; at night it's part of our sleepwear, and in summer we wear it to help prevent dryness and sun damage. It is essential for keeping skin soft and smooth. When you mix in essential oils, your skin gets additional benefits from their anti-ageing, restorative, antioxidant, and skin-softening properties. Use them to make your own beauty-care products – for skin that feels as smooth as silk.

HOW TO USE

Pour a little of the fragrant lotion, cream, or oil into your hand, and apply it to your skin with smooth, sweeping movements, working from your extremities towards your heart: one foot, leg, thigh, buttocks, stomach, then the other foot, leg and thigh, and then the hands and arms. Next, and this is important, wrap yourself in a warm bathrobe, so that the essential oils can do their work.

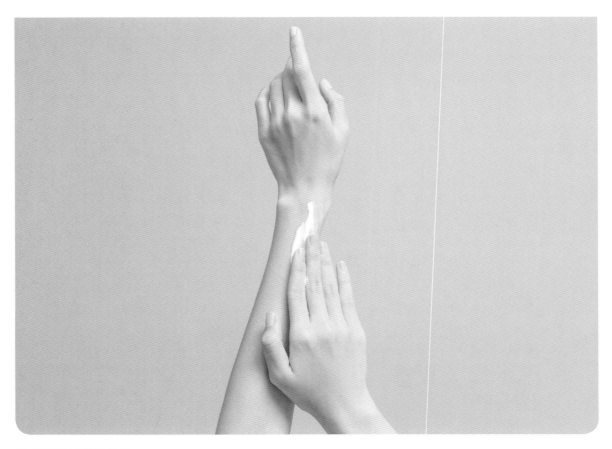

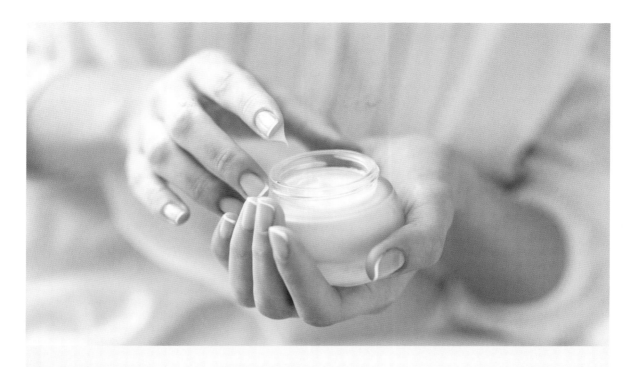

3 BRILLIANT MOISTURIZERS

GORGEOUS OIL FOR A SATIN-SMOOTH SKIN

In a 300 ml (10 fl oz) bottle, mix 5 tbsp argan carrier oil, 5 tbsp apricot kernel carrier oil, 15 drops **lavender essential oil** and 5 drops **lemon essential oil**. Use this only in the evening, as lemon essential oil can increase the skin's sensitivity to the sun.

SUPER REPAIRING BALM

Put ½ tsp white beeswax, 1 tbsp jojoba oil, and 3 tbsp macadamia carrier oil into a heatproof glass jar. Place in a saucepan of water and melt, using the bain-marie method (see page 32), stirring continuously. Take it off the heat, then add 2 tbsp rose hydrolate, then 10 drops **lavender essential oil**, stirring continuously. When all the ingredients are evenly combined, it is ready. This balm can be kept for a month in the refrigerator.

TWO-IN-ONE BALM

Put 5 tbsp shea butter and 2 tbsp argan carrier oil into a heatproof glass jar. Place it in a saucepan of water and melt it, using the bain-marie method (see page 32). Take it off the heat, and slowly add 10 drops **lavender essential oil**, 5 drops **lemon essential oil**, and 5 drops **damask rose essential oil**, stirring continuously. This balm, which will keep for a month in the refrigerator, is also an excellent treatment for dry hair. Use it only in the evening, as lemon essential oil can increase the skin's sensitivity to the sun.

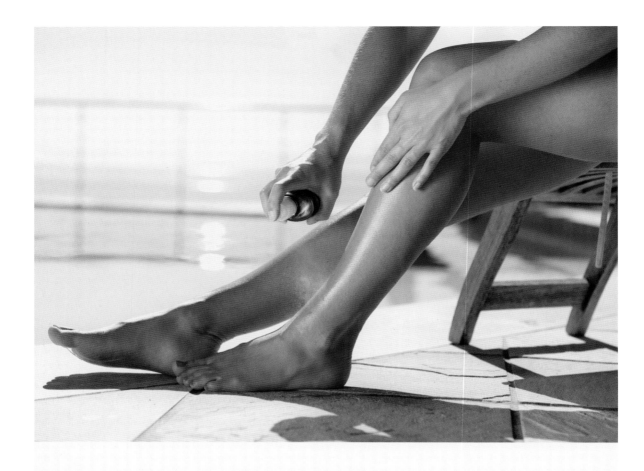

SUN-CARE SOLUTIONS

Of course, everyone now knows the very best way to protect your skin from the sun is – to stay in the shade!

Some people, however, continue to ignore tried-and-trusted health advice; they don't protect their skin from the sun or, at best, they use synthetic products, which may work but are harmful to the planet, and not necessarily good for your health. Sun-care products, prepared at home from essential oils, are not as sophisticated as their shop-bought counterparts, but they are better for the environment and gentler on your skin. For a great tan, protect your skin with natural products, and follow the instructions for safe use – don't spend too long in the sun, avoid the peak hours (midday–4 pm), and wear a hat and sunglasses.

3 BRILLIANT SUN PRODUCTS

BODY-PROTECTING SPRAY

Pour 100 ml (3⅓ fl oz) sesame carrier oil, 200 ml (6¾ fl oz) of jojoba oil, and 5 drops **peppermint essential oil** into a 300 ml (10 fl oz) spray bottle. Use it each time you sunbathe, giving it a good shake before spraying it on your face and body.

HEAT-RASH SOOTHER

Pour 200 ml (6¾ fl oz) lavender hydrolate, 50 ml (1⅔ fl oz) peppermint hydrolate, and 50 ml (1⅔ fl oz) rose hydrolate into a 300 ml (10 fl oz) spray bottle. Shake well and apply twice a day to any inflamed areas of your skin.

REFRESHER SPRAY

Pour 300 ml (10 fl oz) spring water and 6 drops **lavender essential oil** into a 300 ml (10 fl oz) spray bottle. Leave the solution for a week, shaking it once every day. Use the spray on your face, neck, cleavage, and shoulders after each sunbathing session. Shake it well before use, as essential oils do not readily mix with water.

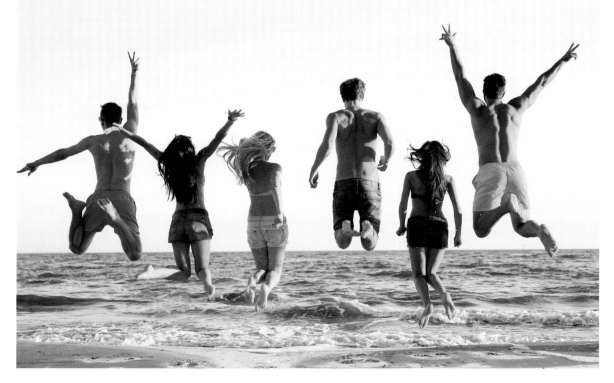

HAND CARE

We ask them to be on duty 24/7, whether it's raining, windy, freezing, or a heatwave, without looking after them. It's no wonder that they are the first to show signs of ageing. It's not too late to put things right. Take advantage of our treatments to give them all the care they need.

METHOD

Apply a little of the balm or oil to the back of each hand, then rub them against each other, as if you were washing them, to spread the product evenly. Then, massage your hands gently, starting from the ends of the fingers and working towards your wrists. Spend a few seconds on each nail.

3 BRILLIANT HAND-CARE PRODUCTS

RAPID HAND SCRUB

In a small bowl, mix 3 tbsp powdered French green clay and 10 drops **lavender essential oil** with a little warm water to make a thick paste. Apply this to the back of the hands once a week, rubbing it in with circular movements. Rinse in clean water.

HAND-IN-GLOVE TREATMENT

In a bowl, mix 1 tbsp olive oil and 6 drops **lemon essential oil**. At bedtime, apply a generous quantity to your hands, then slip on a pair of cotton gloves, and wear them all night. In the morning, rinse your hands in clean water. Try this treatment once a week.

NAIL-STRENGTHENING OIL

In a 10 ml (⅓ fl oz) bottle, mix 20 drops **lemon essential oil** and 8 ml (¼ fl oz) wheatgerm carrier oil. In the evening, slowly massage your nails, one by one, with the mixture, concentrating on the edges and the cuticles. Wipe off with a tissue. Do this once or twice a week.

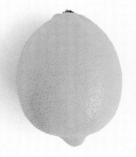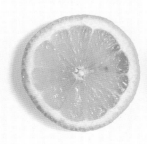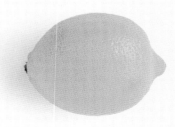

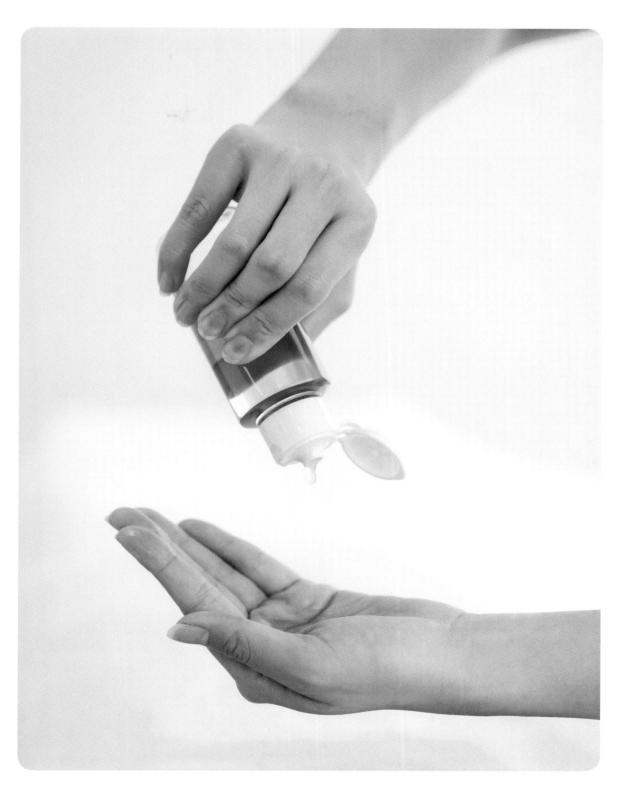

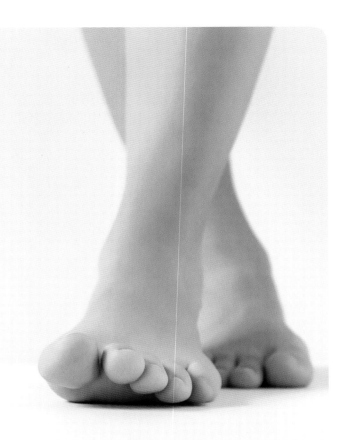

FOOT CARE

Dry, rough, callused soles – imprisoned in footwear, it's all they can do to protect themselves.

Even when we put them in shoes that allow them to breathe, our feet are naturally dry, because of the action of our sebaceous (oil-producing) glands. Moisturizing and nourishing them is essential. Not just so that the skin becomes soft to the touch, but also because then they will carry us further, without reminding us with each step that they are stifling, burning, swelling, and creating corns. The essential oils selected for these treatments all have exceptional properties to help repair even the worst damaged skin.

3 FANTASTIC FOOT TREATMENTS

REFRESHING FOOT CREAM

Melt 4 tbsp shea butter using the bain-marie method (see page 32). Take the pan off the heat and add 5 drops **lemon essential oil** and 5 drops **lavender essential oil**, mixing them well. Wait until the mixture cools, then rub the cream into your feet until it is thoroughly absorbed.

ANTI-BLISTER OIL

Pour ½ tsp sweet almond oil into the palm of your hand. Add 4 drops **tea tree essential oil** and mix together with your finger. Apply the treatment to the chafed areas of your foot, massaging it in well.

BLISSFUL FOOT SCRUB

Add 5 tbsp bicarbonate of soda and 5 drops **rosemary essential oil** to a large bowl of warm water. Stir the water with your hand to mix them, then bathe your feet in the solution for 10 minutes. Take your feet out, but don't rinse them or dry them. Take a handful of bicarbonate of soda and rub it vigorously into the upper side of one foot. Take another handful of bicarbonate and, this time, rub it into the sole and the heel of the foot. Change feet and repeat. Afterwards, rinse your feet carefully with warm water to remove all traces of the bicarbonate.

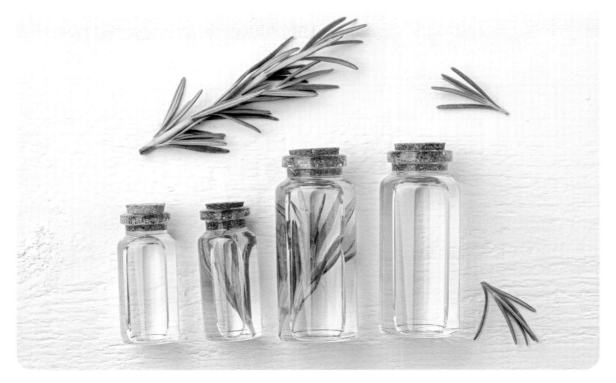

FRAGRANT DEODORANTS

Commercial deodorants have recently come under fire, targeted by the health police for their use of aluminium and parabens, which some studies have linked to cancer.

It's important, however, to do something to curb the smell of perspiration. Essential oils, with their antiseptic properties, come to the rescue yet again to get rid of the bacteria responsible for the odour by natural means.

METHOD

Immediately after washing, carefully dry your armpits and the soles of your feet, then apply the mixture. If you miss the practical application of a roll-on deodorant, worry not; you can buy empty roll-on bottles.

3 GREAT DEODORANTS

FAST DEODORANT CREAM

Take a little of the moisturizing cream you use for your face or body, and mix it with 1 drop **lavender essential oil** and 1 drop **peppermint essential oil**. Stir it with your finger and apply to each armpit.

UNDERARM OR FOOT DEODORANT

Pour a little Isopropyl alcohol 90% into a teaspoon and add 1 drop **peppermint essential oil**. Apply to your feet and/or your armpits with a cotton wool pad.

ULTRA-FRESH FOOT SPRAY

Using an opaque container with a lid or stopper, pour in 40 ml cider vinegar, 20 drops **lemon essential oil**, 20 drops **lavender essential oil**, and 20 drops **peppermint essential oil**. Add 100 ml (3⅓ fl oz) distilled water. Seal the container and shake vigorously to mix the solution. Let it rest for a week, shaking the container once a day, then pour the mixture into a spray bottle. Spray your feet each morning and evening, after washing.

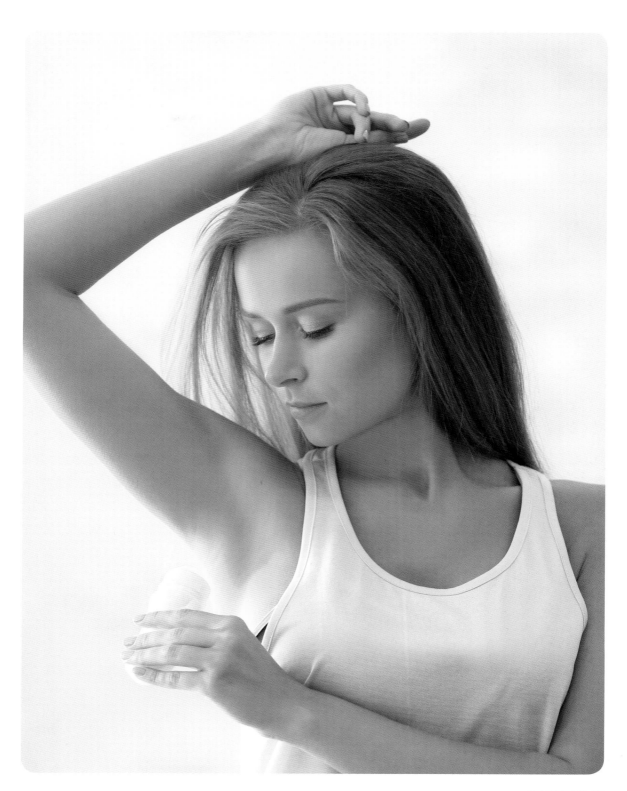

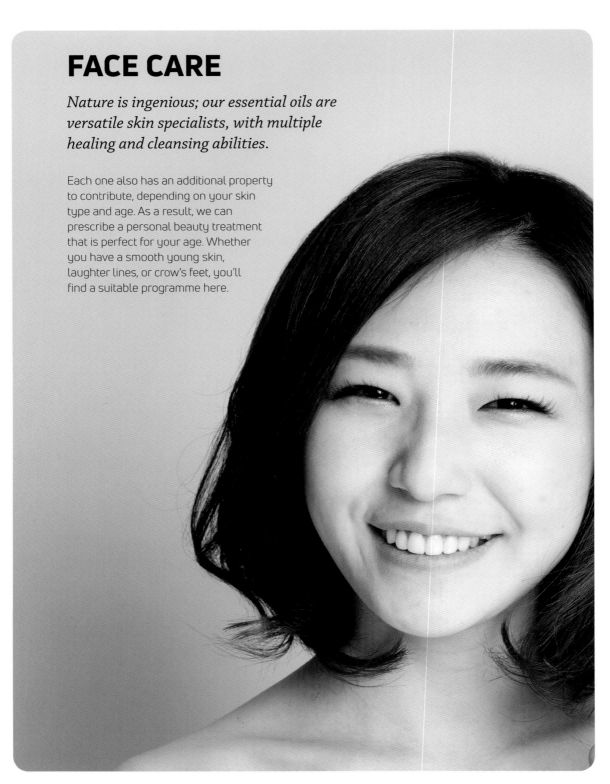

FACE CARE

Nature is ingenious; our essential oils are versatile skin specialists, with multiple healing and cleansing abilities.

Each one also has an additional property to contribute, depending on your skin type and age. As a result, we can prescribe a personal beauty treatment that is perfect for your age. Whether you have a smooth young skin, laughter lines, or crow's feet, you'll find a suitable programme here.

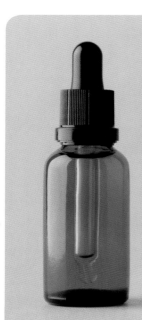

WHICH ESSENTIAL OIL IS FOR YOU?

You have greasy or problem skin. Choose lavender, lemon, tea tree, peppermint, or rosemary cineole.

You have dry or very sensitive skin. Choose lavender.

You have mature skin. Choose damask rose.

IN YOUR TEENS ...

Too young for beauty care, some may say? Looking after your skin from adolescence onwards is an investment in the future. You don't have to spend hours at it, but getting used to ways of nurturing your skin, such as cleansing, exfoliating, moisturizing, and nourishing it, will pay dividends later in life.

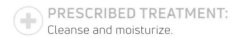 **PRESCRIBED TREATMENT:** Cleanse and moisturize.

SMILEY FACE SCRUB

Pour 1 tbsp orange flower hydrolate, 2 tbsp apricot kernel carrier oil, 1 drop **peppermint essential oil**, and 2 tbsp ground almonds into a bowl, and mix well to create a thick paste. Put a little of the mixture on the tips of your fingers, and apply it to your face and neck, using circular movements and concentrating on the at-risk zones (forehead, nose, and chin). Repeat until you've used up the mixture, then rinse your face in spring water. Dry carefully with a soft towel.

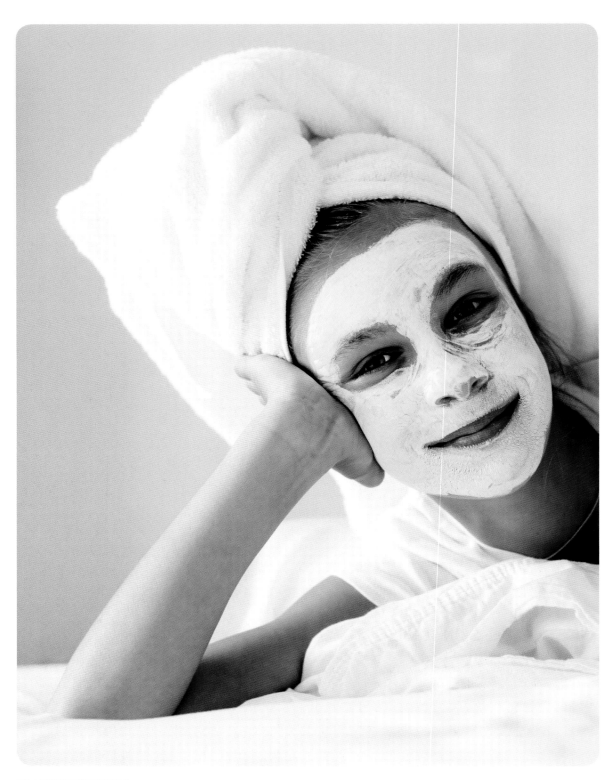

PROBLEM-SOLVING FACE MASK

Pour 3 tbsp powdered French green clay and the juice of ½ lemon into a bowl. Add 3 drops **tea tree essential oil**, 2 drops **peppermint essential oil**, and 1 drop **lemon essential oil**. Mix until you have a smooth paste. Apply the mask in a thick layer, and leave it on for 20 minutes, then rinse it off thoroughly with warm water.

CLEAR SKIN SERUM

Using, if possible, a dark glass bottle with a stopper, pour in 3 tbsp jojoba carrier oil, 5 drops **lavender essential oil**, and 5 drops **rosemary cineole essential oi**l. Shake well to mix the solution. Pour 3 to 4 drops into the palm of your hand, rub your palms together, then apply to clean skin morning and night, massaging from the centre of your face outwards until it has been completely absorbed.

NIGHT OIL

Every evening, before going to bed, quickly prepare this oil: in the palm of your hand, mix together 2 ml apricot kernel carrier oil, 1 drop **damask rose essential oil**, and 1 drop **lavender essential oil**. Apply to a clean face, massaging in small circular movements.

REHYDRATING CREAM

In the palm of your hand, mix together a little aloe vera gel, 2 drops jojoba carrier oil, and 1 drop **lavender essential oil**. Apply it to a clean face first thing in the morning as a day cream, or in the evening, as a night cream.

MAKEUP-REMOVING LOTION

Pour 5 tbsp aloe vera gel, 5 tbsp organic whole milk, and 3 drops **lavender essential oil** into a clean bottle. Shake well, then pour a little of the mixture onto a cotton wool pad. Cleanse your face carefully, and don't worry about getting the lotion on your hair, as aloe vera is good for it. This lotion can be kept for a week in a refrigerator.
CAUTION This makeup-removing lotion should be used only on your face, not your eyes.

LEMON-ROSE LIP BALM

Melt 15 g (½ oz) shea butter in a small saucepan, using the bain-marie method (see page 32). Take it off the heat, then mix in 1 drop **lemon essential oil** and 2 tsp rose hydrolate. Stir, allow to cool, and pour into a small, airtight pot.

GENTLE SKIN TONIC

Using a little 10 ml (⅓ fl oz) atomizer spray bottle, pour in 3 tbsp lavender hydrolate, 3 tbsp rose hydrolate, 2 tbsp cider vinegar, and 5 drops **tea tree essential oil**. Shake well before use and make sure that your skin is free of all makeup.

IN YOUR TWENTIES ...

Your cells still renew themselves with record-breaking speed, your skin is radiant, and the softest it will ever be. But your hidden enemies are on the prowl and advancing: too much sun, too many late nights, junk food, vestiges of makeup, and flare-ups of problem skin are a ticking time-bomb. You need a plan to fight them off.

 PRESCRIBED TREATMENT:
Take control, cleanse your skin, and protect it against free radicals.

A NEAR-PERFECT FACE SCRUB

Mix together 2 tbsp acacia honey with 1 tbsp rye flour, 1 egg yolk, and 3 drops **lavender essential oil** in a bowl. Stir until you have a smooth paste. Apply to your face and neck with the tips of your fingers, using circular movements. Leave the scrub on for 10 minutes, then rinse it off with lemon water (a solution of half water, half lemon juice). Be careful. Use the scrub no more than once a week, and apply a rich skin cream afterwards.

PURIFYING FACE MASK

Mix 2 tbsp honey with 1 tbsp plain fromage frais in a small bowl. Add 2 drops **tea tree essential oil** and 2 drops **rosemary cineole essential oil**, then stir well. Apply this face mask in a thick layer over your forehead, nose, and chin. Leave it on for a quarter of an hour, then rinse it off with lemon water (half water, half lemon juice). Do this twice a week.

BEAUTIFYING SKIN SERUM

Using, if possible, a coloured glass bottle, pour in 3 tbsp argan carrier oil, 1 tbsp apricot kernel carrier oil, and 5 drops **lavender essential oil**. Shake well to mix it. Pour 3 or 4 drops into the palm of your hand, rub your palms together, and apply the preparation to clean skin morning and night, massaging from the middle of your face outwards until it has all been absorbed.

OLD-FASHIONED SKIN TONIC

Put 25 g (⅘ oz) dried rose petals into a jar. Add 300 ml (10 fl oz) rose hydrolate, 50 ml (1⅔ fl oz) cider vinegar, and 2 drops **damask rose essential oil**. Close the jar, and leave it for three weeks away from heat and sunlight. Filter it, and pour it into a little spray bottle. Spray it on a cotton wool pad, and apply after cleaning your face.

MAKEUP-REMOVING LOTION

Pour 250 ml (8½ fl oz) whole milk into a bowl, and add 25 g (⅘ oz) ground almonds and 1 drop **damask rose essential oil**. Stir, leave for an hour, then filter the solution through a thin muslin or a coffee filter. In a well-sealed container, this mixture will keep for a week in the refrigerator. **CAUTION This makeup-removing lotion should be used only on your face, not your eyes.**

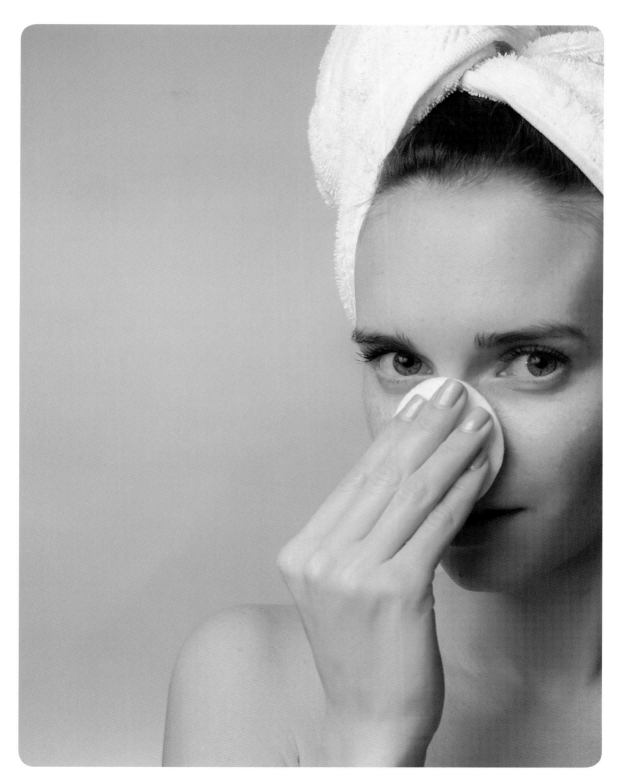

IN YOUR THIRTIES ...

On the plus side, you're all grown up. You can look back to yourself at 20 and agree that you now feel much more comfortable in your skin.

A 30-year-old can think of herself as a real woman, just out of that awkward time between adolescence and adulthood. On the minus side, although you have excellent skin, stress, worries, and pregnancies, too, perhaps, can leave their mark, encouraging the first fine lines.

 PRESCRIBED TREATMENT:
Rejuvenate, moisturize, nourish, and protect your skin. Use face scrubs to encourage exfoliation, and regular face massages to keep the skin firm.

EXFOLIATING FACE SCRUB
Mix 2 tbsp rolled oats, ½ pot natural yogurt, a pinch of salt, and 3 drops **lemon essential oil**. Massage a little of the mixture into your face, concentrating on your forehead, nose, and chin, but avoid the areas around your eyes and mouth. Repeat until you have used up the preparation. To avoid irritating your skin, do this no more than once a week.

OXYGEN MASK
In a small bowl, mix 2 drops **peppermint essential oil,** 3 drops **damask rose essential oil**, and 50 g (1¾ oz) clay paste. Dampen your face with a cotton wool pad dipped in rose hydrolate, then apply the mask in a thick layer. Leave on for 10 minutes, then rinse off with warm water.

REJUVENATING OIL
Using a tinted glass bottle, pour in 60 ml (2 fl oz) argan carrier oil, 40 ml St John's wort infused oil, and 10 drops **damask rose essential oil**. Apply in the morning to a clean face. Store the bottle away from heat and sunlight.

ARABIAN NIGHTS OIL
Pour 6 drops **damask rose essential oil**, 3 drops **lemon essential oil**, and 30 ml (1 fl oz) argan carrier oil into a bottle with a stopper. Shake well before use, and apply each evening to clean skin, massaging it gently in.

CITRUS TONIC
In a bottle with a stopper, mix 300 ml (10 fl oz) orange flower hydrolate, 2 drops **lavender essential oil**, 2 drops **lemon essential oil**, and 10 drops of a natural dispersant or solubilizer. Shake well to mix. In the evening, soak a cotton wool pad in the oil, and apply to clean skin.

FLORAL LIP BALM
Melt 3 tbsp shea butter in a small saucepan, using the bain-marie method (see page 32). Take the pan off the heat, and mix in 2 drops **lavender essential oil** and 2 drops **damask rose essential oil**. Stir, allow to cool, then pour into an airtight jar.

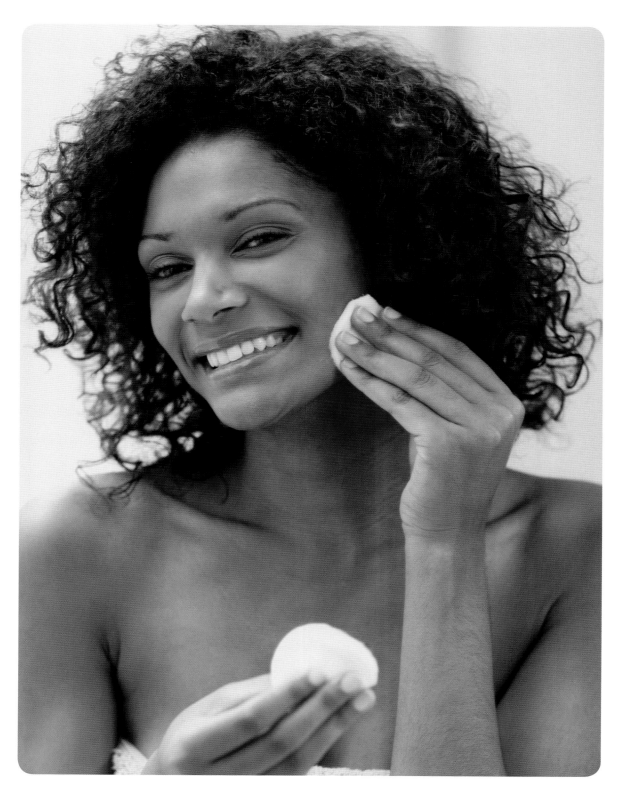

IN YOUR FORTIES …

The very best age to be! (Which, of course, could be said of any age, depending on our lives.) Some women are still not sure what they want from life, but they certainly know by now what they don't want.

That sort of confidence is apparent in the way we dress, our hairstyle, or makeup. Everything would be perfect in the best of all possible worlds, if only signs of ageing weren't involved. Skin is drier, lines settle in, the skin tone is less even, and marked, perhaps, by too much exposure to the sun. The area around the eyes is more crinkled. The good news is that there are a thousand ways to beautify your complexion.

 PRESCRIBED TREATMENT:
Strengthen and stimulate your skin, making its tone more even. Nourish and rejuvenate it. Use a face scrub once a week and a moisturizer every day.

YIN AND YANG FACE SCRUB
Grind 3 tbsp rolled oats to a powder. Add 1 tbsp sweet almond carrier oil and 3 drops **lavender essential oil**. Scoop up a little on the tips of your fingers, and apply to your face and neck, using small circular movements. Repeat until you have used up the mixture, then rinse your face in spring water or lavender hydrolate.

BALANCING FACE MASK
Mix 1 tbsp shea butter with 4 drops l**avender essential oil**. Spread the mask on your face in a thick layer, avoiding the area around your eyes and lips. Leave for 10 minutes, then clean off with a cotton wool pad soaked in lavender hydrolate.

WHIPPED FACE MASK
Beat together 1 egg yolk, 1 tbsp musk rose carrier oil, and 1 tbsp evening primrose oil. Add 1 tsp acacia honey and 3 drops **damask rose essential oil**. Apply to the face, neck and cleavage, leave for 20 minutes, then rinse off with cotton wool soaked in rose hydrolate.

PLUMPING SERUM
Using a 60 ml (2 fl oz) bottle, mix together 2 tbsp borage carrier oil, 2 tbsp evening primrose oil, and 4 drops **damask rose essential oil**. Pour 3 to 4 drops into the palm of your hand, rub your palms together, and apply to your face morning and evening, massaging from the centre outwards until it is fully absorbed.

VODKA TONIC
Pour 100 ml (3⅓ fl oz) rose hydrolate, 4 tbsp lemon juice, 1 tbsp vodka, and 2 drops **peppermint essential oil** into a glass bottle, and shake well. Leave for a day and a night, then use cotton wool to apply it to your face and neck.

PLUMPING LIP BALM

Warm 1 tsp shea butter, using the bain-marie method (see page 32). Take it off the heat, and add 8 drops **lavender essential oil**. Mix well, pour into a small pot, and let it cool.

EYE SERUM

Pour 2 tsp musk rose carrier oil, 2 tsp tamanu (calophyllum) oil, 1 drop **damask rose essential oil**, and 1 drop **lavender essential oil** into a small, glass bottle. Shake well. After cleansing your skin, apply 1 drop of the serum under each eye, morning and evening, massaging very gently from the inside to the outside of the under-eye area. This serum will keep for 3 months if stored in dark place.

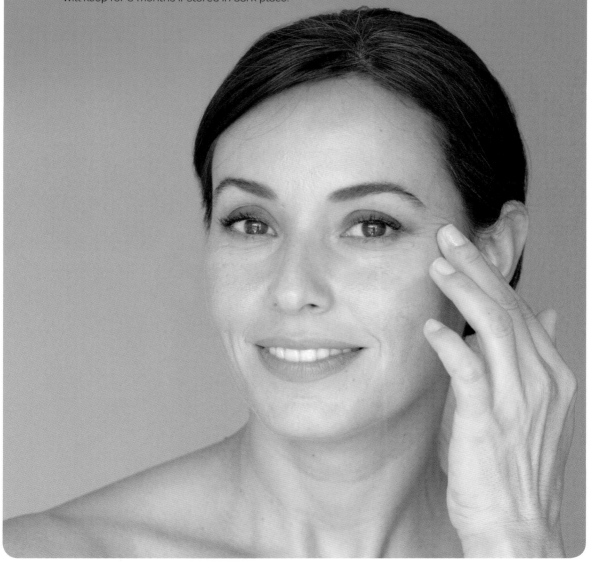

IN YOUR FIFTIES ...

You're wrestling with hormones and everything is shaky. Skin loses its tone, gains lines, and matures. Facial skin begins to sag, wrinkles multiply, and gravity exerts its downward force. That, however, is the catastrophic scenario for those who've done nothing to look after their skin. By contrast, for others it's time to reap the rewards of all that past beauty-care work.

 PRESCRIBED TREATMENT:
Strengthen your skin, boost skin cell renewal, even out your skin tone, and nourish your skin.

SUN SCRUB
Mix 1 tsp powdered coconut with 1 tbsp acacia honey and add 2 drops **lavender essential oil**. Apply to the nose, chin, and forehead, massaging it in, using small circular movements. Rinse with warm water.

REJUVENATING MASK
Mix 1 tsp shea butter, melted using the bain-marie method (see page 32), ½ tbsp borage carrier oil, and 4 drops **damask rose essential oil**. Apply a thick layer of the mixture to your face, avoiding the eye and lip areas. Leave for 10 minutes, then rinse off with cotton wool soaked in rose hydrolate.

LINE-ERASING FACE MASK
Crush around 10 ripe raspberries in a bowl. Add 1 tbsp crème fraîche, 1 tbsp powdered milk, 1 tbsp wheatgerm carrier oil, and 5 drops **lemon essential oil**. Mix well, then apply a thick layer to your face and neck. Leave on for a quarter of an hour, then rinse with lemon water (half water, half lemon juice).

HYDRATING SERUM
Pour 3 tbsp jojoba carrier oil, 1 tbsp musk rose carrier oil, and 5 drops **damask rose essential oil** into a 60 ml (2 fl oz) bottle with a stopper. Each morning, pour 4 drops of the mixture into your palm, rub your hands together, then apply to your skin, moving from the middle of your face outwards until it is fully absorbed.

ROSE-TINGED TONIC
Pour 3 tbsp rose hydrolate into a small bowl, add 3 drops **damask rose essential oil** and 20 drops of a natural dispersant. Shake well. Soak some cotton wool in the solution, and dab it on your face and neck without rubbing. Leave it on for 5 minutes, and don't rinse before applying your regular face cream.

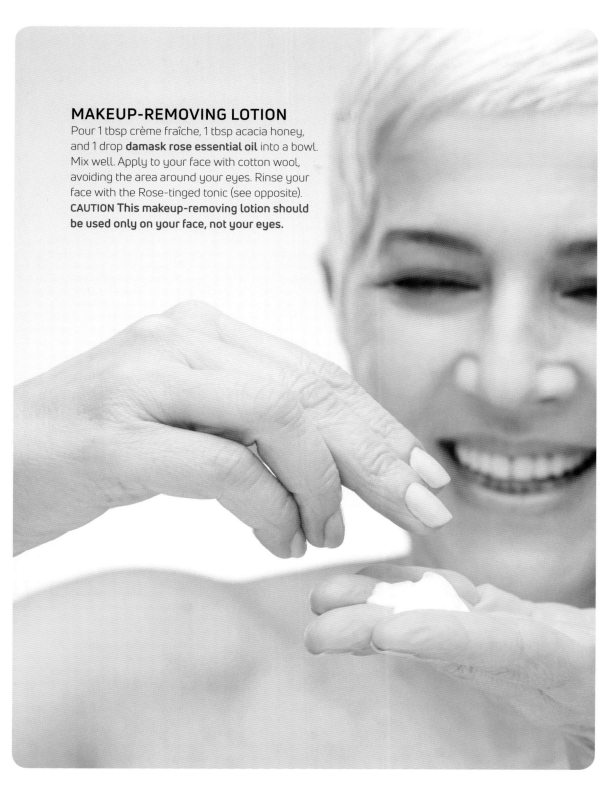

MAKEUP-REMOVING LOTION

Pour 1 tbsp crème fraîche, 1 tbsp acacia honey, and 1 drop **damask rose essential oil** into a bowl. Mix well. Apply to your face with cotton wool, avoiding the area around your eyes. Rinse your face with the Rose-tinged tonic (see opposite).
CAUTION This makeup-removing lotion should be used only on your face, not your eyes.

IN YOUR SIXTIES – AND BEYOND ...

You're embarking on a new life. You're less stressed, more serene, and you have more available time. You'll benefit even more from the moments you spend on beauty care. However, your skin can become much drier and lose its softness. Facial lines deepen, and sun spots begin to appear on your hands, your cleavage, and your face. Quick –essential oils to the rescue!

PRESCRIBED TREATMENT:
Restore and strengthen your skin, combat dehydration, stimulate skin cells at the deepest level, and nourish your skin.

SKIN-REVIVING SCRUB
In a mixer, finely grind 3 tbsp rolled oats, and add 1 tbsp evening primrose oil and 2 drops **damask rose essential oil**. Scoop up a little of this mixture with the tips of your fingers, and apply it to your face and neck, using small circular movements. Repeat until you have used up the mixture, then rinse it off with spring water or rose hydrolate.

ZEN MASK
Mix 1 tbsp aloe vera gel and 4 drops **lavender essential oil.** Spread it in a thick layer on your face, avoiding the areas around your eyes and lips. Leave it on for 10 minutes, then rinse it with cotton wool, soaked in rose hydrolate.

ROSACEA-COMBATING MASK
Before applying your night cream, mix 2 tsp sweet almond oil and 10 drops **lemon essential oil**. Apply the solution, lightly massaging it in, after cleansing your skin. Leave for 30 minutes, then rinse off with lemon water (in a 10:1 solution of water and lemon juice).

MAKEUP-REMOVING LOTION
Pour 2 tbsp jojoba carrier oil, 4 tbsp aloe vera gel, 1 tbsp rose hydrolate, and 3 drops **lavender essential oil** into an atomizer bottle. Shake well before use, then pour a little onto some cotton wool, and apply to your face.
CAUTION This makeup-removing lotion should be used only on your face, not your eyes.

GREEN TEA TONIC
Heat 250 ml (8½ fl oz) water to simmering point. Add 1 tsp of green tea, and allow to infuse for 10 minutes. Strain, then pour it into a bottle with a stopper. Add 1 tsp liquid honey and 4 drops **lavender essential oil**. Shake well. Soak a cotton wool pad in the solution, and apply to clean skin morning and night. This tonic will keep for ten days in the refrigerator.

SUN-SPOT ERASING LOTION

Mix together 10 drops **lemon essential oil**, 10 drops **tea tree essential oil**, and 30 ml (1 fl oz) musk rose carrier oil. Massage your face with the solution, using small circular movements. Keep it for evening use, as lemon essential oil can increase the skin's sensitivity to the sun.

REJUVENATING BALM

Warm ½ tsp beeswax, 1 tsp sweet almond carrier oil, and 1 tsp cocoa butter over a gentle heat, using the bain-marie method (see page 32) and stirring constantly. Take off the heat, then add 1 drop **peppermint essential oil** and 2 drops **lavender essential oil**, still stirring continuously. Pour into a small pot, and keep in the refrigerator.

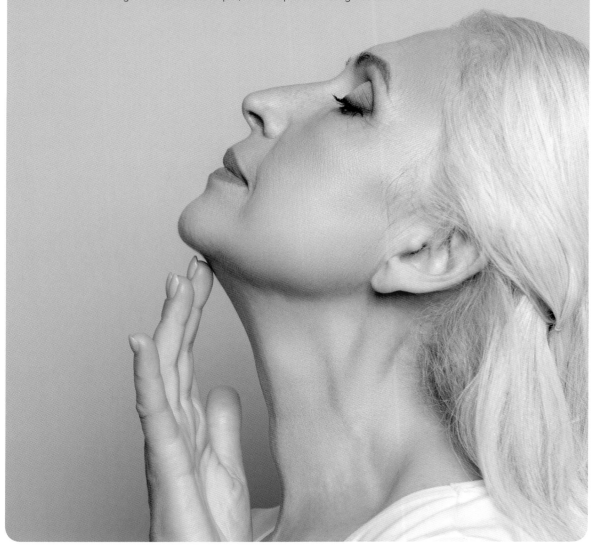

HAIR CARE

You have to get to the root of the problem. All types of hair, whether dry, greasy, dull, sparse, or falling out, can be treated with an appropriate essential oil. Once you find the right one, your hair will become more beautiful and will benefit from its natural protection. It's a chance for you to create a shampoo, mask, or lotion that perfectly matches your hair's needs.

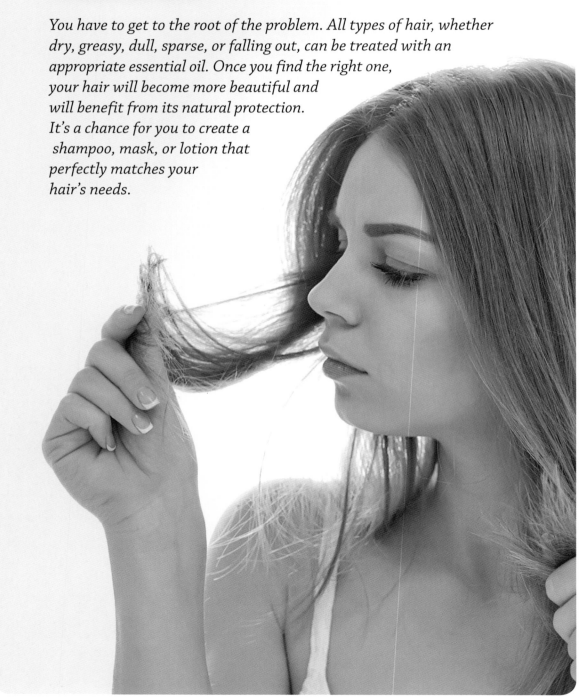

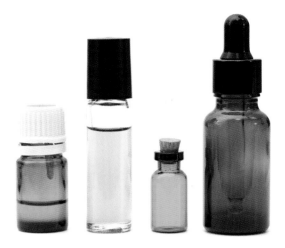

FRAGRANT HAIR MASKS

METHOD

- Masks should be applied to dry hair. Mix the essential oils with 100 ml (3⅓ fl oz) carrier oil, and apply to the roots, parting your hair into layers, as you would when using a tint. Pour whatever remains onto the rest of your hair, massaging it in to ensure it is well absorbed.
- Wrap your hair in some cling-film, tie a warm towel over it, and leave for 15 minutes.
- Then shampoo your hair as normal, and rinse well afterwards.
- Repeat the process once a week.

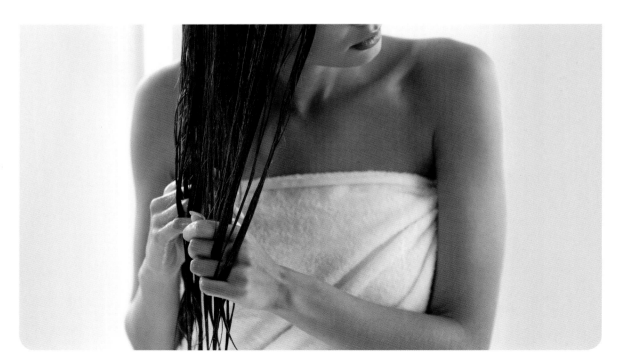

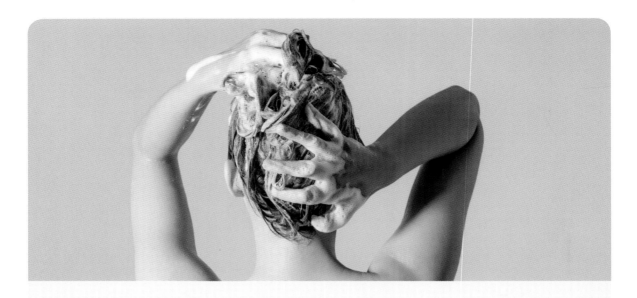

FRAGRANT SHAMPOOS

METHOD
- A fragrant shampoo has remarkable constituents, but is used quite simply. Like a normal shampoo, you should apply it to damp hair, massaging it in well with your fingertips.
- Leave the shampoo on for 5 minutes, then rinse off in plenty of water. The bravest finish with an almost cold rinse.

3 BRILLIANT SHAMPOOS

TO COMBAT HAIR LOSS
Pour 10 drops **rosemary cineole essential oil** and 10 drops **lemon essential oil** into a 500 ml (17 fl oz) bottle of neutral shampoo (sold online and in stores that sell organic products). Shake well before each use.

FOR DRY HAIR
Pour 10 drops **lavender essential oil**, 10 drops **rosemary cineole essential oil**, and 1 tbsp safflower carrier oil into a 500 ml (17 fl oz) bottle of neutral shampoo. Shake well before each use.

FOR GREASY HAIR
Pour 5 drops **lavender essential oil** and 10 drops **lemon essential oil** into a 500 ml (17 fl oz) bottle of neutral shampoo Shake the bottle well before each use, and avoid over-hot water which stimulates the sebaceous glands.

FRAGRANT LOTIONS AND CONDITIONERS

Whether or not we have highlighted or tinted hair, we're all hooked on our conditioners. Without them, hard water can leave hair coarse and difficult to untangle. But synthetic smoothing products can sometimes do more harm than good.

2 GREAT LOTIONS AND CONDITIONERS

CONDITIONER FOR NORMAL HAIR

Beat together 1 egg yolk, 1 tsp glycerine (available from pharmacies or online), 2 drops **rosemary cineole essential oil**, and 3 drops **lavender essential oil**. Add 1 tbsp powdered milk, and mix to a smooth cream. Apply this to damp hair, after you've rinsed it, massaging your scalp with your fingertips. Leave on for 5 minutes, then rinse in warm water. A final rinse with a cider vinegar solution (see below) will make your hair shine and get rid of any of the limescale in hard water that dulls hair.

A SHINING HAIR RINSE (ALL HAIR TYPES)

Pour 2 glasses of cider vinegar, 10 drops **lavender essential oil** and 5 drops **lemon essential oil** into a 1 litre (2 pint) glass bottle. Fill up with spring water and shake well to mix. When you have washed and rinsed your hair, pour half a glass of this solution into 1 litre (2 pints) warm water, and use this for your last rinse.

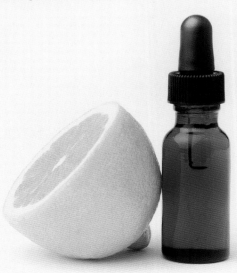

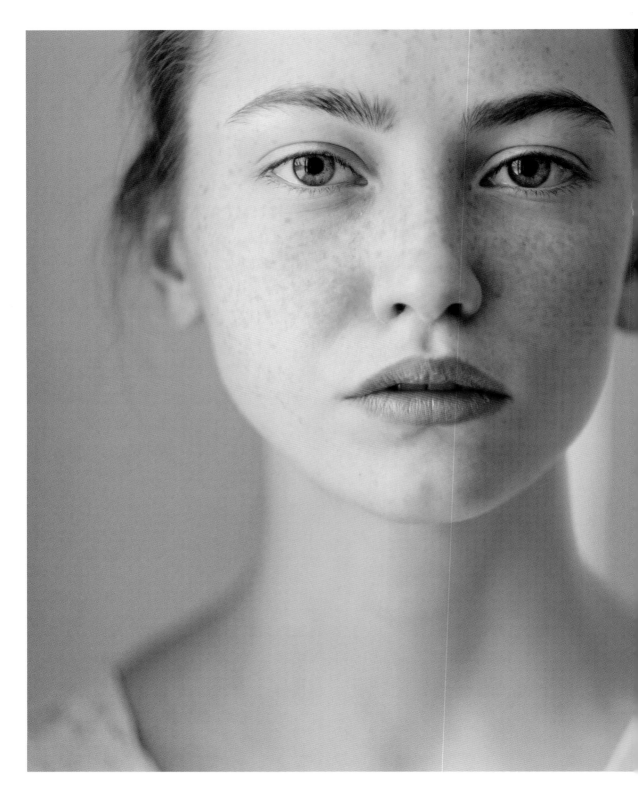

LOOKING AFTER MIND AND BODY

Whether the problem is acne, cuts, bumps, colds, or insomnia, you'll see how effective these six brilliant essential oils are for treating everyday ills. Prepare to be very surprised by the results of using these natural 'medicines'. They act quickly and well, without you having to worry about side effects, when they are used correctly. The essential oils that we have chosen cover the majority of ills that can make everyday life miserable. They are multi-talented, and just a few drops may treat a viral infection, or freshen the air, or help boost poor circulation. But don't get carried away. Essential oils are powerful, and it isn't a question of improvising. The dosages recommended here are precise and must be observed.

COMMENTS

- Essential oils are not designed to be long-term treatments. Without exception, you should follow the advice until symptoms disappear and for no more than five consecutive days, if taking by mouth.
- Essential oils act very rapidly. If you don't get clear results within the indicated time, don't persist with them. You may not have diagnosed the problem correctly and may not be using the appropriate essential oil. Take advice.
- Advice regarding the ingestion of oils varies from country to country. It is advisable to consult a qualified aromatherapist before using remedies marked with an asterisk*.

MENTAL WELL-BEING

ANXIETY
• Rub two drops **lavender essential oil** on to the insides of your wrist and breathe in the fragrance whenever you need to.

NERVOUS EXHAUSTION
• Open a bottle of **peppermint essential oil**, and breathe in its fragrance calmly and deeply several times a day.
• *Add 1 drop **peppermint essential oil** to ½ tsp honey, and let the mixture melt in your mouth. Repeat as necessary.

TIREDNESS
• Mix 20 drops **peppermint essential oil**, 20 drops **rosemary cineole essential oil**, and 2 tsp hazelnut carrier oil in a small bottle. Massage your temples with the oil (avoiding your eyes), then rub it vigorously on your forearms and calves.
• Pour 10 drops **lemon essential oil**, 3 drops **peppermint essential oil**, and 5 drops **rosemary cineole essential oil** into a diffuser, and diffuse the mixture in your living area for 1 hour in the morning and in the afternoon.

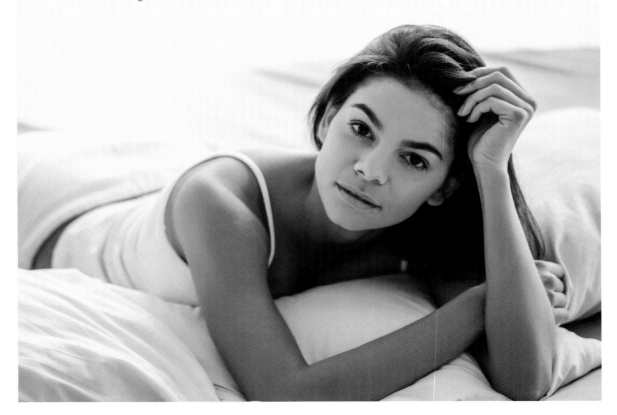

NEURASTHENIA (CHRONIC FATIGUE SYNDROME)

- Inhale the fragrance of **damask rose essential oil** straight from the bottle as often as you need to.

INSOMNIA

- *Add 2 drops **lavender essential oil** to 1 tsp honey, and mix it into a lime-blossom tisane. Drink 1 cup after dinner and 1 cup before going to bed.
- Spray several drops of **lavender essential oil** on your pillow as you go to bed. It will help you relax – and keep mosquitoes away.
- Mix 20 drops **lavender essential oil** and 1 tbsp bath oil base. When you've run a warm bath, pour in this mixture and soak in the water (heated to about 38°C/100.4°F) for 20 minutes. Don't rinse it off, and quickly tuck yourself up in a cosy bed.

EMOTIONAL SHOCK

- If someone has just received upsetting news that induces a state of shock, pour 2 drops **peppermint essential oil** onto a handkerchief. Breathing in its aroma will bring relief.

DIZZINESS LINKED TO STRESS

- Mix 4 tbsp of coarse grey salt, 20 drops **lavender essential oil**, and 10 drops **peppermint essential oil** in a bottle. When you feel dizzy, reach for your salts, and breathe deeply from the bottle.
- Mix 10 drops **lavender essential oil** and 5 drops **peppermint essential oil** with 1 tbsp bath oil base. When you've run a warm bath, pour in the mixture, and soak in the water (heated to about 38°C/100.4°F) for 20 minutes.

ANGER

- Sprinkle 2 drops **lavender essential oil** on a handkerchief, and breathe its fragrance as often as necessary.

DEPRESSION

- Diffuse **lavender essential oil** in the rooms you live in several times a day. Continue until the depression lifts.

SEASONAL AFFECTIVE DISORDER

- Diffuse 10 drops **lemon essential oil** in your living areas for 10 minutes twice a day.

FEELING LOW

- Put 1 drop **peppermint essential oil** on each wrist, and breathe in its aroma three or four times a day.

BAD MOOD

- Pour 2 drops **lavender essential oil** and 1 drop **peppermint essential oil** onto a handkerchief. Breathe in their fragrance two or three times a day.

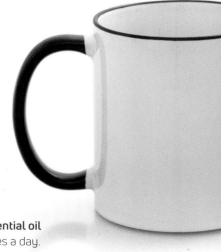

NERVOUSNESS
• Apply 1 drop **lavender essential oil** to your temples whenever you need it.

APHRODISIAC
• Use a diffuser of **damask rose essential oil** in your bedroom for 10 minutes in the evening, or breathe its perfume straight from the bottle twice a day for ten days.

SEXUAL FATIGUE
• Inhale from a bottle of **damask rose essential oil** every evening for three weeks.

MEMORY
• To boost your memory, diffuse 5 drops **rosemary cineole essential oil** and 5 drops **lemon essential oil** in your office for 10 minutes twice a day.

CONCENTRATION
• Put 1 drop **rosemary cineole essential oil** on each wrist, and breathe it in deeply every time you need to.

CONCENTRATION WHEN DRIVING
• *Put 1 drop **lemon essential oil** on your tongue every 2 hours. Alternate with coffee or other stimulant drinks.

TIREDNESS WHEN DRIVING
• If you have to drive for a long time, every hour, diffuse a few drops **peppermint essential oil** in a car diffuser, plugged into your cigarette lighter. That will keep you awake and alert, and reduce your tiredness levels.

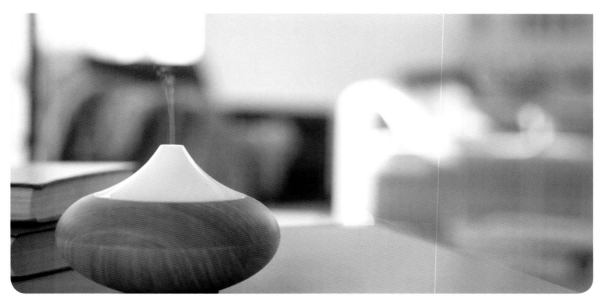

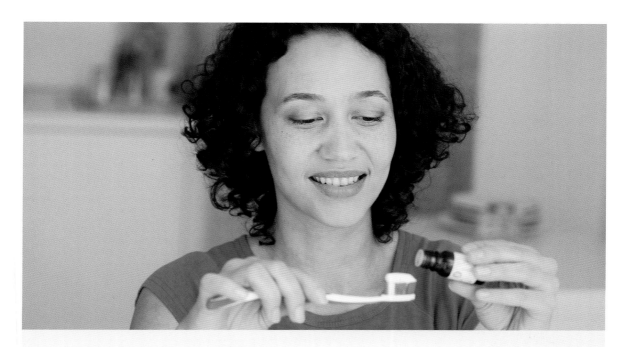

MOUTH CARE

TOOTH ABSCESS
- During the course of the day, apply 1 drop **peppermint essential oil** and 1 drop **tea tree oil** alternately to the gum around the painful area, using cotton buds.

MOUTH ULCER
- Rinse your mouth with a solution of 5 drops **tea tree essential oil** diluted in ½ glass of warm water. Repeat three times a day.

DENTAL HYGIENE
- Twice a week, pour 2 drops **tea tree essential oil** onto your toothbrush before you squeeze out the toothpaste.

BAD BREATH
- Pour 2 drops **peppermint essential oil** into a small glass of water. Rinse your mouth with it before spitting it out. This mouthwash will refresh your mouth for several hours. Use it after each meal.

ORAL THRUSH
- Apply 2 drops **tea tree essential oil**, diluted with 2 drops calendula infused oil, to the affected area, using your finger or a cotton bud. Do this three to five times a day until the symptoms disappear.

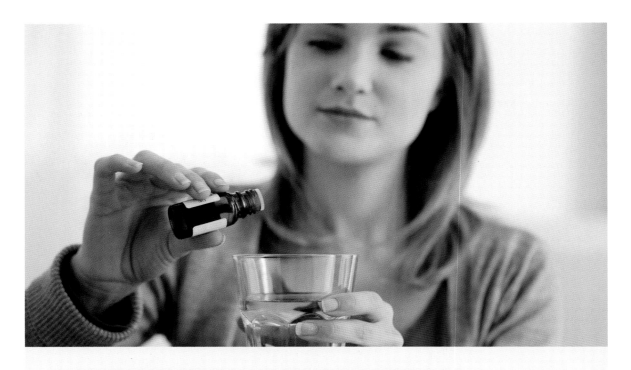

CIRCULATION AND HEART CARE

ROSACEA

- Mix 50 ml (1⅔ fl oz) tamanu (calophyllum) oil and 10 drops **lemon essential oil**. Ensure that your face is perfectly clean, then lightly massage in the solution. Let your skin absorb it for half an hour, then rinse it off with lemon water (1 part lemon juice to 10 parts water), before you apply your night cream.

HIGH BLOOD PRESSURE

- *Add 2 drops **lavender essential oil** to 1 tsp honey, then mix with ½ glass of water. Take this two or three times a day.
- Apply 2 drops **lavender essential oil** three times a day to your solar plexus (just above your navel), to the inside of your wrists, and to the arch of your foot.

LOW BLOOD PRESSURE

- Mix 5 drops **rosemary cineole essential oil** with 3 drops **peppermint essential oil** in 2 tsp hazelnut carrier oil. Massage your body with this mixture once a week.
- *Add 2 drops **peppermint essential oil** to 1 tsp olive oil, and take twice a day, preferably in the morning and at midday, not in the evening.

PAIN

ARTHRITIS
- Mix 2 drops **peppermint essential oil**, 3 drops **lavender essential oil**, and 5 drops arnica infused oil. Massage the painful areas with this mixture three times a day.

MUSCLE STRAINS
- Apply 4 to 5 drops **lavender essential oil** to the painful muscle, gently massaging it in.

SPRAINS
- Add 2 drops **peppermint essential oil** and 3 drops **lavender essential oil** to a bowl of iced water. Lay a thin cloth on the surface of the liquid to absorb the oils. Wring out the cloth, and apply it to the sprain for 15 to 20 minutes.

HEADACHES
- Soak a handkerchief in very cold water, sprinkle it with several drops of **lavender essential oil** and **peppermint essential oil**, then apply to your forehead, keeping it away from your eyes. Renew it as often as required.
- *Add 1 drop **peppermint essential oil** to 1 tsp honey, mix this into a cup of regular or herbal tea, and drink it.
- Diffuse a few drops of **lavender essential oil** and **peppermint essential oil**, preferably using an electric diffuser, for 10 minutes in living areas, such as your bedroom and office.

MUSCLE SPASM
- Apply 4 to 5 drops **lavender essential oil** to the painful muscle and massage gently.

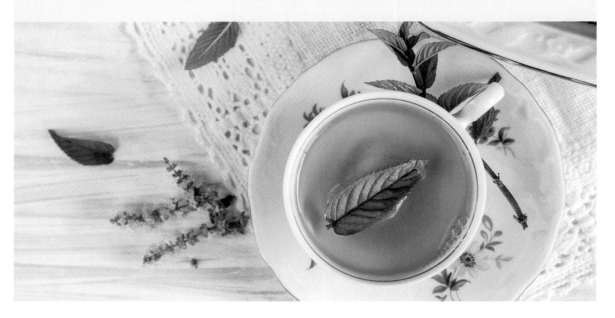

PREGNANCY

USING ESSENTIAL OILS DURING PREGNANCY

Aromatherapy, used alone or as an accompaniment to conventional medical treatments, can treat various problems, whether they are associated with pregnancy or not. It can help a pregnant woman regain her emotional equilibrium (which also benefits her unborn child), or control an infection, inflammation, or a circulatory problem, which may or may not be linked to her pregnancy. But be very careful. While pregnant, do not take essential oils by mouth, except perhaps lemon or ginger essential oils, which may help combat morning sickness in the early months, but they should only be taken as advised by a qualified aromatherapist.

CHILDBIRTH (COMBATING PAIN AND STRESS)

- Apply several drops of **damask rose essential oil** to the insides of your wrists, and inhale its perfume as calmly and deeply as possible.

ACNE

- Mix 5 drops **lavender essential oil**, 5 drops **tea tree essential oil**, and 1 tsp musk rose carrier oil. Apply 1 drop of this mixture to the spots, twice a day until they clear up.

FLATULENCE (BELCHING, WIND)

- *Mix 2 drops **lemon essential oil** and 5 drops olive oil in a spoon. Pour it into your mouth, under your tongue, after midday and evening meals. Do this for four to five days, if necessary.

BREASTFEEDING (STOPPING)

- *Take 2 drops **peppermint essential oil** on a neutral tablet (available online), or with 1 tsp honey, three times a day, allowing it to melt in your mouth.
  CAUTION It is essential to stop breastfeeding before you first take this remedy.

SMALL WOUNDS AND SORES

- Mix 1 drop **lavender essential oil**, 1 drop **tea tree essential oil**, and 2 drops calendula infused oil. After cleaning the area with soap and water, apply this mixture three times a day for two days, then in the morning and evening until it heals.

HAIR LOSS

- Pour 4 drops **lemon essential oil** into your regular shampoo (preferably a clay shampoo).

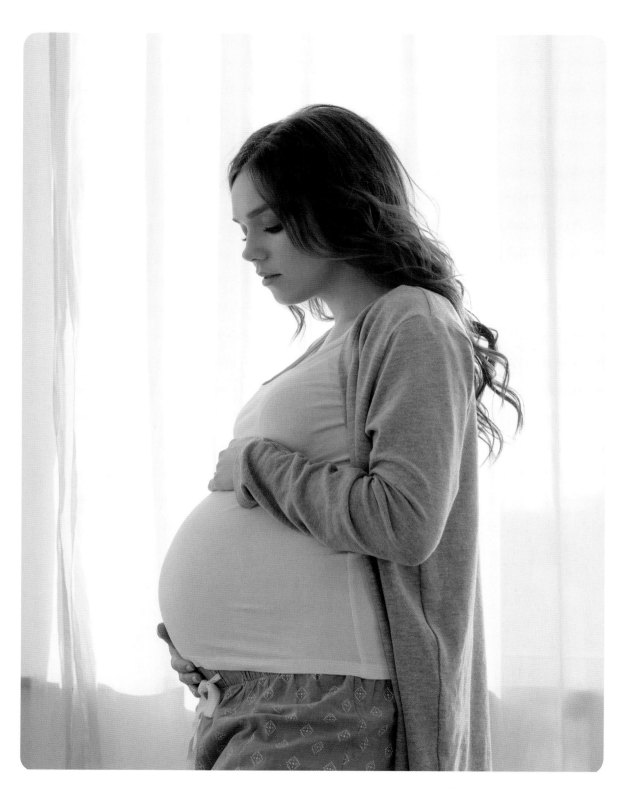

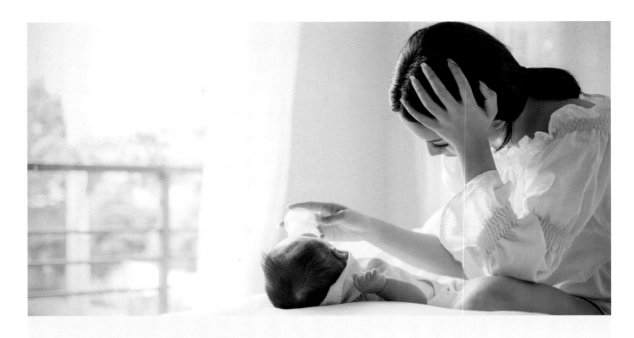

POST-NATAL DEPRESSION

- Mix 1 tbsp apricot kernel carrier oil and 4 drops **damask rose essential oil** in a small bottle. Place 1 drop of the mixture on the inside of your wrists, and inhale its fragrance every time you feel the need to do so.
- Apply 5 drops of the mixture on your solar plexus three times a day, until the symptoms disappear.

LIVER DETOX

DURING PREGNANCY

- *Add 2 drops **lemon essential oil** to ½ tsp olive oil. Let the mixture dissolve in your mouth. Do this three times a day for eight days each month. You can substitute ½ tsp honey for the olive oil, and take the mixture in a cup of tea.

AFTER PREGNANCY

- *Mix 1 drop **peppermint essential oil**, 1 drop **rosemary cineole essential oil**, and 1 tsp honey. Pour the mixture into 500 ml (17 fl oz) rosemary infusion. Drink gradually over 24 hours; do this for eight days.

DIGESTIVE PROBLEMS

- *Mix 1 drop **lemon essential oil** with ½ tsp honey and allow to dissolve in your mouth after a heavy meal.

ECZEMA

- Mix 5 drops **tea tree essential oil**, 5 drops **lavender essential oil**, and 1 tsp evening primrose oil. Gently massage the solution into the affected areas three or four times a day until the symptoms disappear.

CHILBLAINS

- Mix 1 drop **lavender essential oil** with 2 drops musk rose carrier oil. Apply to the affected area three times a day until it has completely healed.

EPISIOTOMY

- Mix 3 drops **lavender essential oil** and 1 tbsp bath oil base in a basin (or bidet) of warm water, and take a sitz bath for 5 minutes, twice a day, until the area heals.
- Mix 2 drops **lavender essential oil** and 2 drops musk rose carrier oil. Apply to the area with your finger three times a day, until it is completely healed.

FLU

- Pour 10 drops **lemon essential oil** into a diffuser. Diffuse the mixture for 10 minutes, three times a day.

INSOMNIA

- Pour 10 drops **lavender essential oil** into your diffuser, and diffuse for 15 minutes in your bedroom at bedtime.
- Pour a few drops **lavender essential oil** on your pillow.

LOW LIBIDO

- Apply 1 drop **damask rose essential oil** on your solar plexus and 1 drop on the inside of each wrist, then inhale deeply, morning and evening, until you notice some improvement.
- Mix 1 ml **damask rose essential oil** and 9 ml (³⁄₁₀ fl oz) musk rose carrier oil in a small bottle. Ask your partner to massage your spine with a few drops of this mixture in the evening.
- Inhale the fragrance of **damask rose essential oil** direct from an open bottle, three to four times a day.

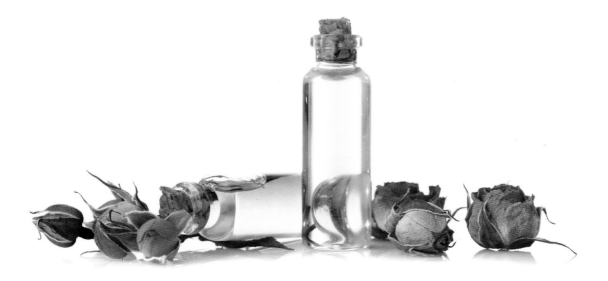

HEADACHE
- Pour 10 drops **lavender essential oil** into your diffuser, and diffuse for 10 minutes.

TRAVEL SICKNESS
- *Pour 1 drop **lemon essential oil** into ½ tsp honey, and allow it to dissolve in your mouth, as often as necessary during a journey.

NAUSEA
- *Pour 2 drops **lemon essential oil** into ½ tsp honey, and hold the mixture in your mouth, letting it dissolve, before you get up.
- *Pour 2 drops **lavender essential oil** into ½ tsp honey, and let the mixture melt in your mouth. Do this as often as you need to.

WATER RETENTION
FROM THE 4TH MONTH OF PREGNANCY
- *Pour 1 drop **lemon essential oil** into ½ tsp honey or olive oil, and let the mixture melt in your mouth. Do this three times a day for four to five days.

EXCESS WEIGHT
FROM THE 4TH MONTH OF PREGNANCY
- *Place 1 drop **lemon essential oil** under your tongue, allowing it to melt in your mouth. Do this three times a day.

SHINGLES
- Mix 1 drop **tea tree essential oil**, 1 drop **lavender essential oil**, and 5 drops St John's wort infused oil. Apply the mixture to the blisters up to eight times a day.

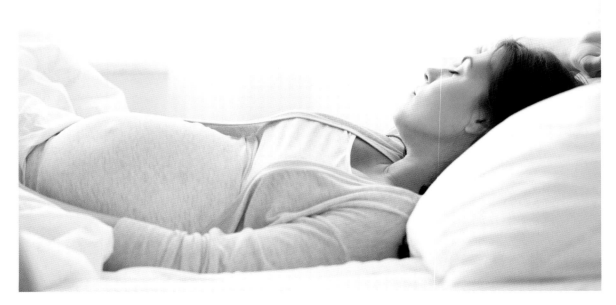

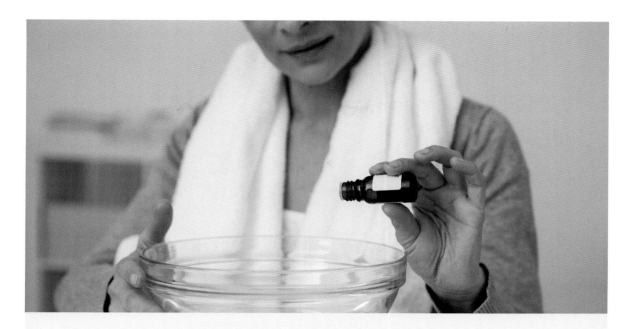

EAR, NOSE, AND THROAT PROBLEMS

SORE THROAT
- *Dilute 1 drop **tea tree essential oil** in 1 tsp honey, and allow to melt in your mouth. Do this two to three times a day. Alternatively, add the mixture to an aromatic herbal tea, such as thyme, rosemary, or sage, and drink two to three times a day.
- Dilute 1 drop **peppermint essential oil** and 2 drops **tea tree essential oil** with 1 tbsp acacia honey. Add this to a half glass of warm water. Stir well, and gargle with the mixture three times a day for three days.

QUITTING SMOKING
- Mix 20 drops **lemon essential oil** and 20 drops **peppermint essential oil** in a small bottle. Each time you feel like smoking, reach for the bottle instead, and inhale the fragrance of these essential oils.

BRONCHITIS
- Pour 6 drops **tea tree essential oil** into a bowl of hot water, and inhale the steam for 10 minutes, twice a day.
- Use an electric diffuser to diffuse 8 drops **lemon essential oil** in your living areas for 20 minutes in the morning and evening.

WHOOPING COUGH
- Dilute 2 drops **rosemary cineole essential oil** in 1 tsp sweet almond carrier oil, and massage the lung area two or three times a day.

FEVER AND INFECTIONS (BABIES AND CHILDREN)

- To calm a child: gently massage the solar plexus and the insides of the wrists with 2 drops **lavender essential oil** diluted in several drops of sweet almond carrier oil several times a day.
- To treat disorders such as colic, infections, and sleep problems, massage the stomach area several times a day with 2 drops **lavender essential oil** diluted in 1 tsp sweet almond carrier oil.

FLU

- Mix 4 drops **tea tree essential oil**, 4 drops **lemon essential oil**, and 2 tsp macadamia carrier oil. Using 10 drops of this mixture, gently massage the neck, chest, and top of the back four times a day, until the symptoms subside.

RESPIRATORY INFECTION

- Apply 2 drops **tea tree essential oil** to the chest area and top of the back four times a day for ten days.
- *Add 1 drop **tea tree essential oil** to 1 tsp honey, and let it melt in your mouth. Do this four times a day for ten days.

LARYNGITIS

- Dilute 1 drop **peppermint essential oil** and 2 drops **tea tree essential oil** in 10 drops hazelnut carrier oil. Apply the mixture around the ear area and on the neck three times a day, keeping well away from the eyes.

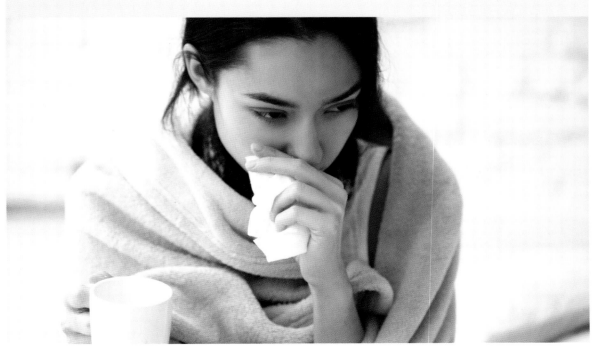

CONGESTED NASAL PASSAGES

- *Put 1 drop **peppermint essential oil** under the tongue. If necessary, do this two or three times a day.

MUMPS

- Dilute 2 drops **tea tree essential oil** in a little sweet almond carrier oil, and apply three times a day around the ears, jaw, and neck. Do this for five days.

EAR INFECTION

- Mix 1 drop **lemon essential oil** and 1 drop **tea tree essential oil**. Massage a little of the mixture around the ear. Do this three times a day until symptoms subside.
  OR, if the ear is not weeping:
- Soak a little ball of cotton wool in the solution, and place it in the painful ear. Renew as often as necessary until it feels better.

HEAD COLD

- Apply 2 drops **tea tree essential oil** four times a day to the nostrils, throat, and chest area for two to three days.
- *Dilute 2 drops **tea tree essential oil** in ½ tsp honey, and let this melt in your mouth. Do this four times a day for two to three days.

HAY FEVER

- Pour 200 ml (6¾ fl oz) water, 10 drops **lavender essential oil**, and 5 drops **peppermint essential oil** into a spray bottle. Shake well, then spray in your living areas two or three times a day.

SINUSITIS

- Pour 4 drops **tea tree essential oil** and 2 drops **peppermint essential oil** into a bowl of hot water, and inhale the steam for 10 minutes twice a day. Don't go out for 2 hours after the treatment.
- Mix 6 drops **tea tree essential oil** and 2 drops **peppermint essential oil** in 2 tsp hazelnut carrier oil. Using 10 drops of the mixture, gently massage the forehead and sinus areas on each side of the nose two or three times a day.

CHESTY COUGH

- Mix 4 drops **tea tree essential oil**, 4 drops **rosemary cineole essential oil** and 2 tsp hazelnut carrier oil. Using 8 drops of the mixture, rub your chest and the top of your back twice a day until symptoms disappear.
- *Place 1 drop **tea tree essential oil** under your tongue, and let it melt in your mouth. Do this four times a day.

DRY COUGH

- Pour 2 drops **rosemary cineole essential oil** and 2 drops **peppermint essential oil** onto a handkerchief, and breathe in their fragrance as often as necessary.

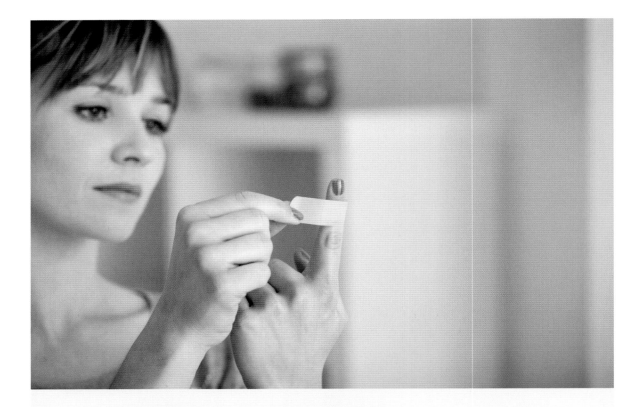

SKIN PROBLEMS

ABSCESS
• Apply 1 drop **tea tree essential oil** directly to the abscess under the dressing three times a day for five days.

ACNE
• Mix 1 tsp **tea tree essential oil** and 2 tsp apricot kernel carrier oil in a small 15 ml (½ fl oz) bottle. Apply 2 drops of the mixture to the affected areas every morning and evening. Store the bottle out of the light.

PIMPLES AND BOILS
• Mix 5 drops **tea tree essential oil** and 5 drops **lavender essential oil** with 2 tsp calendula infused oil. Apply three times a day to scrupulously clean skin.

CUTS
• Apply 1 drop **lavender essential oil** and 1 drop **tea tree essential oil** to the area three times a day for two to three days. Cover with a dressing.

BURNS AND SCALDS

- Mix 1 tsp **lavender essential oil** and 1 tsp musk rose carrier oil. After cooling the burn or scald under cold water for 5 minutes, apply 3 to 8 drops of this mixture four times a day for three to six days, as required.
- If only a small area is affected, you can apply a few drops of **lavender essential oil** directly. Do this every 10 minutes until the pain subsides.

SCARS

- Mix together 3 drops **lavender essential oil** and 4 drops musk rose carrier oil. Apply this mixture to the scar twice a day for ten days. Gently massage the length of the scar to boost blood circulation and stimulate cell renewal in the affected area.

ITCHING (ANYWHERE ON THE BODY)

- Mix together 3 ml **lavender essential oil**, 1 ml **peppermint essential oil** and 2 tsp calendula infused oil in a small bottle. Apply 3 to 8 drops of this solution (depending on the size of the skin area to be treated) four times a day until the symptoms disappear.

ECZEMA

- Dilute 10 drops **tea tree essential oil** and 10 drops **lavender essential oil** with 1 tbsp bath oil base. Pour into a bath of water, and take a soothing soak for 20 minutes.

SORES

- Wash the sore with soap and water, and rinse it well with clear water. Then apply 2 drops **tea tree essential oil** on and around the wound to clean the whole area and prevent infection. Do this several times a day.

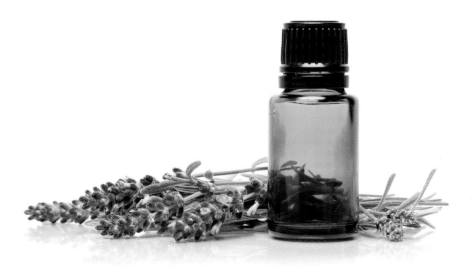

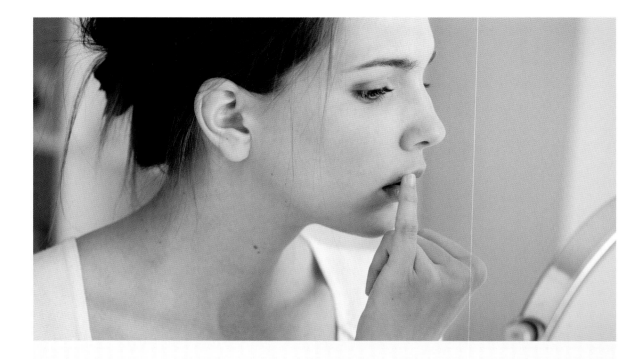

BEDSORES

- **Prevention:** add 50 drops **lavender essential oil** to 250 ml (8½ fl oz) cider vinegar. Using a soft cloth, apply this mixture three times a day to susceptible areas.
- **Treatment:** Mix 6 ml **lavender essential oil** with 4 ml musk rose carrier oil in a small bottle. Apply 6 drops of this mixture on the affected areas four times a day, and allow air to get to the sore for as long as possible, as often as possible.

COLD SORES

- Apply neat **tea tree essential oil** to the affected area with the tip of your finger six to eight times a day for two days, then three times a day until it heals.

IMPETIGO

- Apply 1 drop **tea tree essential oil** to the infected area three times a day for eight to ten days.

CHAPPED LIPS

- Mix together 1 ml **lavender essential oil** and 4 ml musk rose carrier oil in a small bottle. Apply 2 drops of this preparation twice or three times a day until your lips heal.

INGROWN TOENAIL

- Bathe your feet in hot water. Soak a cotton wool pad in 1 tsp olive oil mixed with 3 drops **tea tree essential oil**. Wrap the affected nail in the cotton pad, slip on a sock over your foot, and keep it on all night.

ATHLETE'S FOOT

- Fill a bowl with hot water. Dilute 4 drops **tea tree essential oil** and 3 drops **lavender essential oil** with 1 tsp bath oil base. Pour this mixture into the bowl, stir, and soak your feet in it for 20 minutes. Don't rinse them, but dry them well.
- Mix 2 ml **tea tree essential oil** with 3 ml jojoba carrier oil. After each bath or shower, carefully dry your feet, then apply several drops of the preparation to the affected areas.

INSECT OR ANIMAL BITE

- Apply 1 drop **lavender essential oil** to the bite as soon as possible. Repeat three times a day.

HEAD LICE

- **Prevention** (when there is an outbreak): pour 10 drops **lavender essential oil** into a 250 ml (8½ fl oz) bottle of shampoo, and wash hair as normal.
- **Treatment:** Massage your scalp with a compress soaked in a solution of 5 drops **tea tree essential oil** and 10 drops **lavender essential oil**. Cover your head with a shower cap for the night. Do this for three consecutive days, then repeat eight days later.

TICKS

- Apply 3 drops **tea tree essential oil** to the area. Wait for 5 minutes, then remove the tick with a tick remover (available from a pharmacy or online). Then, disinfect the wound with a further drop of tea tree essential oil. Keep an eye on the area.

WARTS

- Apply 1 drop **tea tree essential oil** directly to the wart and cover it with a little dressing. Repeat the treatment, and renew the dressing each day until the wart disappears.

ANTISEPTICS: WHY ESSENTIAL OILS ARE PREFERABLE TO TRADITIONAL REMEDIES

- **Essential oils** They have both powerful anti-bacterial and healing properties.
- **Isopropyl alcohol** 90% It smarts, irritates, and dries the skin.
- **Camphor spirit** Camphor is potentially toxic and has an irritant action, and is therefore not suitable for cleaning wounds.
- **Tincture of iodine** It has an effective antiseptic action and heals wounds quickly. But traditional iodine preparations tend to smart, dry up the skin, and leave stains.
- **Hydrogen peroxide** It works well but can destroy healthy cells, which can slow healing. Never apply it to compresses that will be left on the skin for a long time.
- **Eosin solution** Its powerful action is mostly used for drying up sores.
- **Ether** It has no antiseptic effect, and its vapour is toxic.

* Availability of the above products may vary from country to country.

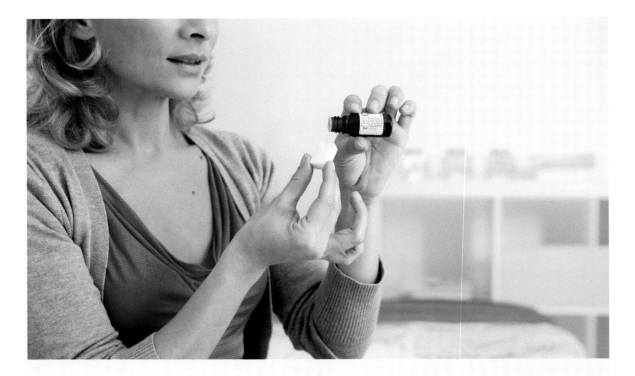

DIGESTIVE SYSTEM

TRAVEL SICKNESS
- *Add 1 drop **lemon essential oil** and 1 drop **peppermint essential oil** to a sugar lump. Let it dissolve in your mouth. Repeat as often as necessary.
- Mix 3 ml **lemon essential oil** and 2 ml **peppermint essential oil** in a small bottle. Before travelling by air, land, or sea, massage your forehead with 2 drops of this solution, and repeat during the journey.

WIND
- *Place 2 drops **peppermint essential oil** under the tongue, and let it melt in your mouth. Do this three times a day.
- Massage your lower stomach area with 2 drops **lavender essential oil** three times a day.

HEARTBURN
- *Add 1 drop **peppermint essential oil** and 1 drop **lemon essential oil** to ½ tsp honey, and take this after a meal. Repeat if necessary.
- Mix together 2 drops **peppermint essential oil** and 10 drops calendula infused oil. Massage your stomach with the mixture after each meal for several days.

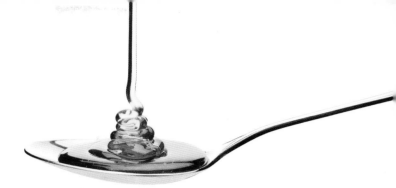

LACK OF APPETITE

- *Dilute 2 drops **peppermint essential oil** in ½ tsp honey, and take this before meals. Continue the treatment for around twenty days.

BILIOUS ATTACK (LIVER PROBLEMS AND NAUSEA)

- *Add 2 drops **peppermint essential oil** to ½ tsp honey, and take after meals. Do this three times a day for three days.

DIARRHOEA

- Massage your stomach three to five times a day with 2 drops **tea tree essential oil**. Do this for two days.

SLOW DIGESTION

- *Dilute 1 drop **lemon essential oil** and 1 drop **peppermint essential oil** in 1 tsp honey. Add the mixture to a hot drink, and take after each meal for several days.

FLATULENCE

- Massage your stomach in a clockwise direction with 2 drops **lavender essential oil** once or twice a day.

GASTROENTERITIS

- *Hold 1 drop **peppermint essential oil** under your tongue four times a day between meals for three days, then three times a day for two days.

HANGOVER

- Pour 2 drops **peppermint essential oil** onto a handkerchief and take deep breaths from it.
- *Pour the juice of ½ lemon into a cup, and fill it with warm water. Add 1 drop **lemon essential oil** diluted in 1 tsp honey, and drink.

VIRAL HEPATITIS

- *Add 2 drops **peppermint essential oil** to ½ tsp honey, and allow to melt in the mouth. Do this three times a day, and continue the treatment for twenty days.

INDIGESTION

- *Add 2 drops **peppermint essential oil** to a neutral tablet (available online), or 1 tsp honey, and let it dissolve in your mouth. Do this three times over the course of 24 hours.

LIVER FAILURE
- *After a meal, take 1 drop **lemon essential oil** and 1 drop **peppermint essential oil** diluted in 1 tsp honey.

MORNING-AFTER FEELING
- *Add 2 drops **peppermint essential oil** to ½ tsp honey and let it melt in your mouth. Repeat as necessary, as often as necessary.

DIGESTIVE FUNGAL INFECTION (CANDIDIASIS)
- *Pour 2 drops **tea tree essential oil** onto a neutral tablet (available online), or 1 tsp honey, and let it melt in the mouth. Do this four times a day for twenty days.

NAUSEA
- Pour 2 drops **peppermint essential oil** onto a handkerchief, and breathe from it each time you feel sick.
- *Add 1 drop **peppermint essential oil** to a neutral tablet (available online), or to 1 tsp honey, and take this several times a day until symptoms subside.

DIGESTIVE SPASMS
- Gently massage the lower stomach with 2 drops **lavender essential oil** three times a day.

STOMACH ULCERS
- *Add 2 drops **peppermint essential oil** to ½ tsp honey, and allow to melt in the mouth. Do this twice a day.

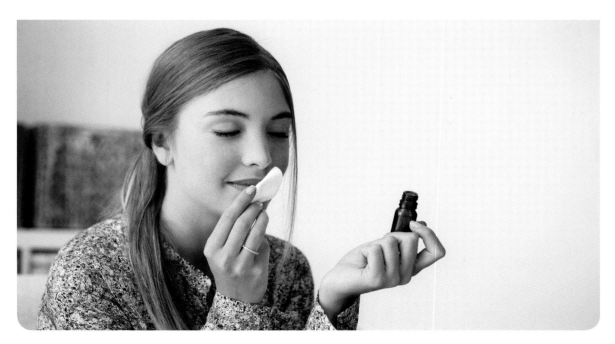

GENITO-URINARY SYSTEM

CYSTITIS
- *Add 2 drops **tea tree essential oil** to 1 tsp honey, and let it melt in the mouth. Do this four times a day for three days.

VAGINAL ITCHING
- Mix 2 drops **tea tree essential oil** and 4 drops calendula infused oil. Apply with your fingertip to the affected area.

FERTILITY (ENCOURAGING)
- Inhale the fragrance of **damask rose essential oil** directly from the bottle, three or four times a day.
- Using 3 drops **damask rose essential oil**, you and your partner should work together gently massaging your solar plexus areas and spine columns. The best time is in the evening when you can relax completely and enjoy your sexual relationship. Continue this for several weeks if necessary.

LOW SEX DRIVE
- Inhale the fragrance of **damask rose essential oil** direct from the bottle.

MENOPAUSE
- When you feel a hot flush coming on, massage your forehead and neck with 1 drop **lavender essential oil**.

THRUSH
- *Add 2 drops **tea tree essential oil** to 1 tsp honey, and take this three times a day for five to seven days.
- Apply 2 drops **tea tree essential oil** to your lower stomach area and lower back four times a day for five to seven days.
- Mix 1 drop **tea tree essential oil** with 5 drops St John's wort infused oil. Apply with your fingertip to the vagina.

WHITE DISCHARGE
- Mix 20 drops **lavender essential oil** with ½ tsp essential oil dispersant or solubilizer. Pour the mixture into 1 litre (2 pints) warm water, and use this in a vaginal douche. Do this in the morning and evening when you wash.

PAINFUL PERIODS
- *Hold 1 drop **peppermint essential oil** under your tongue, and repeat as necessary.

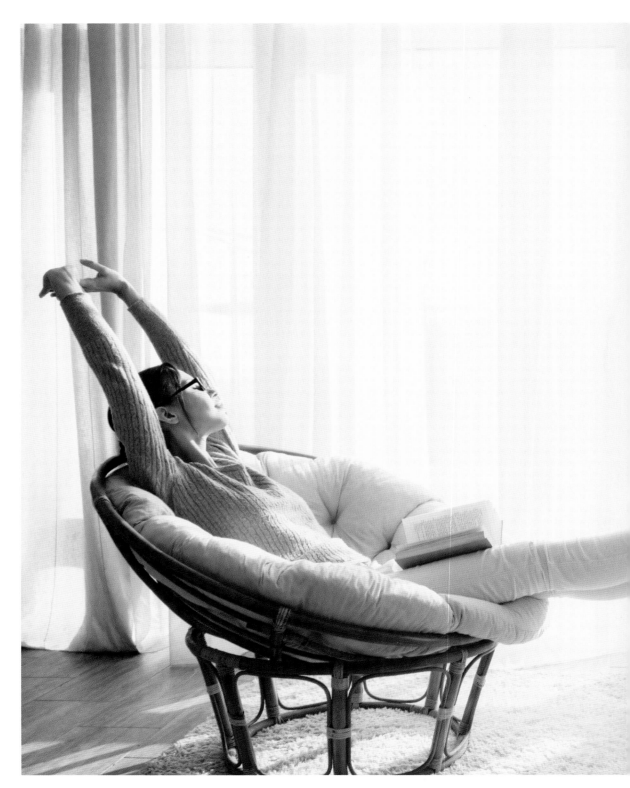

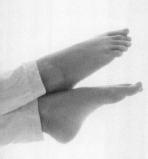

A FRESH, FRAGRANT HOME

Lemon, peppermint, tea tree, rosemary cineole, lavender, and damask rose – our six well-being fairies have antibacterial properties and delightful perfumes. That's all they need to become household magicians, too. A refrigerator that opens with the fragrance of a field of lavender, a bathroom redolent with the fresh scent of lemon, ironing that smells like sweet, rose-flavoured Turkish delight. With these essential oils, housework is enchanting. No polluting, synthetic cleaning agents, no enemies of the planet, and a clean, fragrant home. And to make it as easy as using readymade products, we offer 'recipes' treasured by our grandmothers and great-grandmothers, and handed down the generations. They use traditional ingredients such as bicarbonate of soda, white vinegar, black soap or Marseille soap, natural substances which have been rediscovered in a new, environmentally-conscious age.

THE KITCHEN

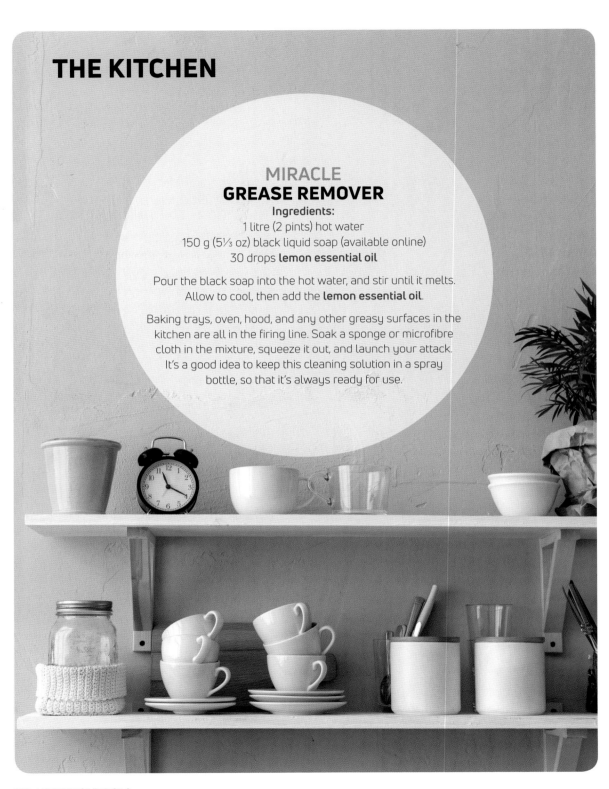

MIRACLE
GREASE REMOVER

Ingredients:
1 litre (2 pints) hot water
150 g (5⅓ oz) black liquid soap (available online)
30 drops **lemon essential oil**

Pour the black soap into the hot water, and stir until it melts.
Allow to cool, then add the **lemon essential oil**.

Baking trays, oven, hood, and any other greasy surfaces in the
kitchen are all in the firing line. Soak a sponge or microfibre
cloth in the mixture, squeeze it out, and launch your attack.
It's a good idea to keep this cleaning solution in a spray
bottle, so that it's always ready for use.

CLEANSING AIR-FRESHENER

Roasts, fry-ups, grills – they're wonderful! But, once you've cleared away the dishes, the residual smells are less appetizing and can become quite nauseating. Pour 10 drops **lavender essential oil** and 10 drops **lemon essential oil** into a diffuser. Diffuse for 20 minutes – time enough for a little stroll, which will do you good, after everything you've eaten.

AIR-FRESHENER 2

A diffuser is the best way of using essential oils to freshen a room, especially when there are colds and flu around, for example. However, if you don't have one, you can recycle a 300 ml (10 fl oz) spray bottle, pouring in 250 ml (8½ fl oz) spring water and 20 drops **lemon essential oil**. Shake well before spraying the room.

SPONGES

Sponges are a haven for bacteria and bad smells. They often end up burned by bleach or in the bin, because you haven't found a less aggressive or sweeter-smelling cleaning product. Instead, fill a bowl three quarters full of water, add 3 drops **lemon essential oil**, and soak the sponge in it. Wring it, then put it in the microwave on maximum power for 30 seconds.

SEALS

To safeguard the seals on the doors of your refrigerator, washing machine, and dishwasher, and treat (or prevent) brown mildew stairs, the ideal solution is **tea tree essential oil**. Pour a few drops onto a sponge, and wipe over the seals, leaving the solution on for a few minutes, before rinsing it off with cold water.

DISHWASHER

Should you wash your dishwasher? No, but you should keep it fresh and free of smells. Pour 40 drops **rosemary cineole essential oil** into a 200 ml (6¾ fl oz) spray bottle, then top up with white vinegar. Shake the bottle, and spray the dishwasher twice a week.

SUPER-EFFECTIVE WASHING-UP LIQUID

Using a small funnel, pour 8 tbsp black liquid soap, 1 tbsp bicarbonate of soda, 1 tbsp white vinegar, and 20 drops **lemon essential oil** into a 500 ml (17 fl oz) clean, empty washing-up liquid bottle. Close the lid, and shake vigorously to ensure they're well mixed. This is a very concentrated solution, so you'll only need one squirt for dishes from a meal for four. Don't forget to shake the bottle before each use.

MICROWAVES

Pour 3 drops **peppermint essential oil** or **lemon essential oil** into a bowl of water. Microwave for 2 or 3 minutes on full power. Wait for about 10 minutes before taking out the bowl to ensure you have got rid of the smells of all the various dishes you have cooked in it. Use the same mixture to sponge over and clean the interior of the microwave.

PANTRY MOTHS (INDIAN MEAL MOTHS)

They can appear any time of year, usually at night – dull-coloured, idling, little moths. But the harm has already been done. They've laid their eggs everywhere possible, including packets of cereal, flour, and rice, which their larvae feed on. You'll have to sort everything out, throwing away affected foodstuffs, and storing untouched foods in sealed jars. Then, you should vaccuum your cupboard shelves and clean them with this mixture: 1 glass of white vinegar and 5 drops **peppermint essential oil,** mixed into a bowl of hot water.

MILDEW

It starts with a humid film on surfaces, which then turns black. And it can happen almost anywhere; for instance, on walls, in corners, or at the bottom of shower curtains. Don't let mildew appear; get rid of it with your faithful allies. Pour 300 ml (10 fl oz) hot water, 100 ml (3⅓ fl oz) white vinegar and 5 drops **tea tree essential oil** into a spray bottle. Shake to mix the solution. Spray the affected areas, clean with a fresh sponge, dry with a clean cloth, then lightly spray them again.

WASTE BIN

Before your put your bin bag into the waste bin, throw in a piece of cotton wool or kitchen roll dipped in 4 drops **lemon essential oil**. That's one solution for two problems: the lemon will combat both bacteria and unpleasant smells.

REFRIGERATOR

Pour 500 ml (17 fl oz) hot water, 500 ml (17 fl oz) white vinegar, and 3 drops **lemon essential oil** into a small basin. Soak a sponge or microfibre cloth in the solution, and carry out a thorough clean of all shelves and compartments. Leave the door open, so that it dries.

Next, pour 2 drops **lemon essential oil** onto a piece of porous stone (such as pumice), and place it in a compartment in your fridge door. To maintain the fresh smell, recharge your pumice stone regularly with the essential oil.

STEAMING, ROSEMARY-SCENTED, ROLLED TOWELS

Here's a classy touch to end the Asian meal you've prepared. And not just Asian dishes: the custom of presenting guests with hot, rolled towels at the end of a meal is also very welcome after mussels or other seafood.

Pour 250 ml (8½ fl oz) rose hydrolate and 250 ml (8½ fl oz) spring water into a bowl. Soak inexpensive little squares of terry cloth (available online) in the solution, then wring them out. Then, pour a little of the solution into a steamer, and add 6 drops **rosemary cineole essential oil**. Fold and roll the squares of cloth tightly, and place them in the top part of the steamer. Cover, and set to boil for 5 minutes. Take out the rolled towels with tongs, and bring immediately to the table on a little tray.

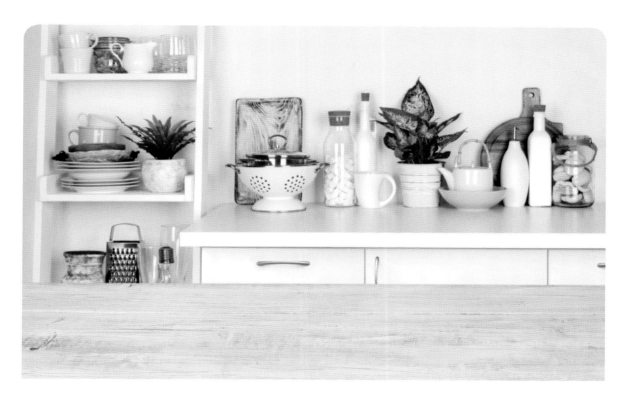

LIQUID SOAP

It's well known that there's nothing better than lemon for getting rid of the smell of fish or garlic. This soap, which blends the deodorizing effect of lemon with the perfume of lavender, will do a brilliant job. Pour 100 ml (3⅓ fl oz) neutral liquid soap, 15 drops **lemon essential oil**, and 15 drops **lavender essential oil** into a pump spray bottle. Shake well to blend the mixture.

FLOORS

A two-in-one solution that disinfects floors and leaves behind a gentle scent of lavender is surely appealing. Pour 1 tbsp black liquid soap, 2 drops **lemon essential oil**, and 2 drops **tea tree essential oil** into a bucket of very hot water. It is best to use a self-wringing, microfibre mop, so you don't have to put your hands in the solution, and, unlike regular mops, it won't leave any messy residue.

SCENTED COASTERS

Without becoming an avid coaster collector, you could get together some decorative, or even vintage, beer mats, to protect your coffee table. If you like the idea, pour 1 drop **lemon essential oil** on each one at tea or coffee time; when you place a hot drink on them, they will give off a delicate lemon fragrance.

THE LAUNDRY

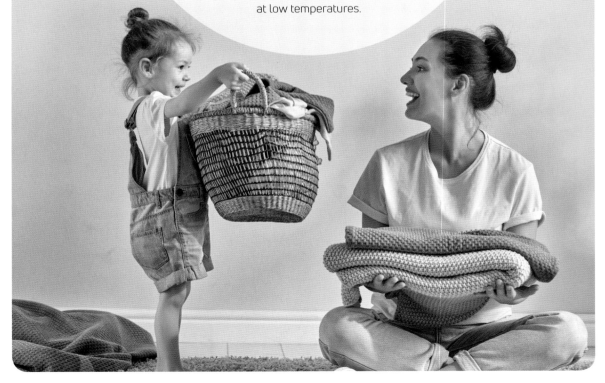

MIRACLE
LAUNDRY DETERGENT

Ingredients:

3 litres (6⅓ pints) water

150 g (5¼ oz) Marseille soap

10 drops **tea tree essential oil**

Grate the soap, and spoon it into a large, clean, empty detergent container, then add 3 litres (6⅓ pints) boiling water. Shake vigorously to dissolve the soap, then add the **tea tree essential oil**.

Before each use, shake the container to mix the detergent, then add 200 ml (6¾ fl oz) of the solution to the detergent compartment of your washing machine. This 100 per cent natural, homemade detergent delights the senses; it protects your laundry from germs, and has a clean and fresh scent, thanks to the Marseille soap. With this detergent, there is no risk of allergies, and it works well even when washing at low temperatures.

A SUPERSOFT FABRIC CONDITIONER

Mix 500 ml (17 fl oz) white vinegar and 1 tsp **lavender essential oil** in a strong plastic or glass bottle with a cap. Mark its contents clearly on the outside. When you're about to wash a load of laundry, shake the bottle well, and pour about 100 ml (3⅓ fl oz) into the conditioner compartment of your washing machine. Always shake the bottle before use.

The vinegar will keep your laundry soft and fresh, and will also remove any limescale traces that can make material coarse. It brightens white fabrics, too, and gets rid of perspiration marks, and any odours. At the same time, it prolongs the life of your washing machine by removing limescale each time you use it. Use your favourite essential oil; whichever one you choose, its fragrance will outshine that of the fanciest synthetic product.

IRONING WATER

Add 3 drops **lavender essential oil**, or **peppermint essential oil**, or **damask rose essential oil** to the water in your steam iron. There's no risk of staining fabrics as essential oils are not greasy. However, you should perhaps avoid using it when you iron shirts and blouses as your own perfume might clash with the fragrance of lavender, peppermint, or rose.

TUMBLE-DRYER SHEETS

When you're about to start tumble-drying your laundry, pick out a cloth, a napkin, or a sock. Pour 10 drops **lavender essential oil** onto whichever one you've chosen, and tumble-dry it with the rest. The oil will add its fragrance to all your garments, without staining or damaging them. Even better, you will not be using any non-recyclable dryer sheets!

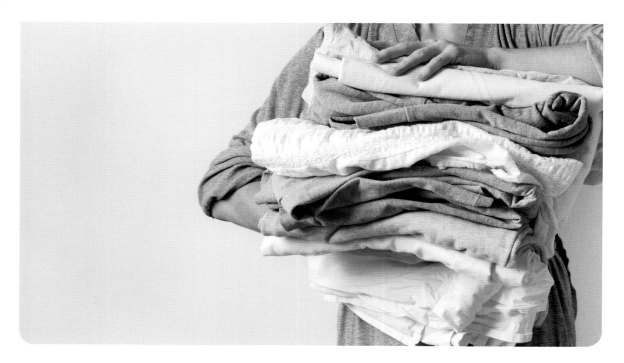

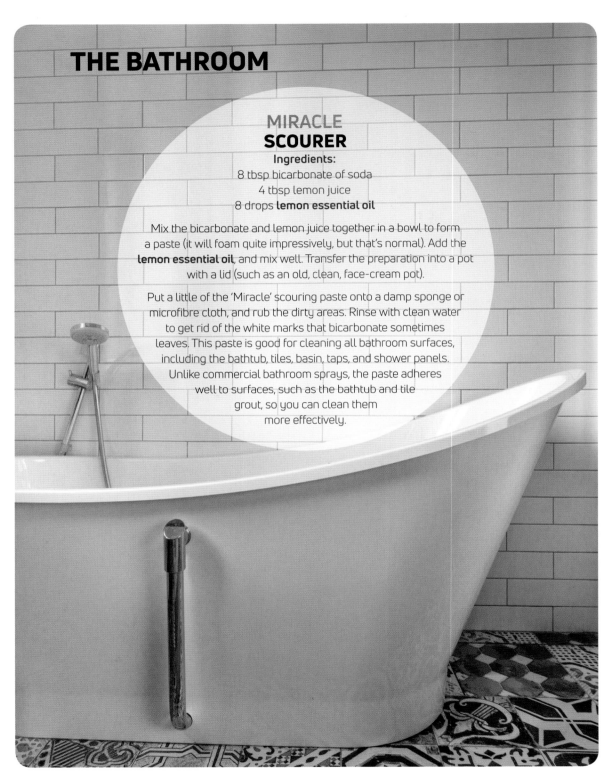

THE BATHROOM

MIRACLE
SCOURER

Ingredients:
8 tbsp bicarbonate of soda
4 tbsp lemon juice
8 drops **lemon essential oil**

Mix the bicarbonate and lemon juice together in a bowl to form a paste (it will foam quite impressively, but that's normal). Add the **lemon essential oil**, and mix well. Transfer the preparation into a pot with a lid (such as an old, clean, face-cream pot).

Put a little of the 'Miracle' scouring paste onto a damp sponge or microfibre cloth, and rub the dirty areas. Rinse with clean water to get rid of the white marks that bicarbonate sometimes leaves. This paste is good for cleaning all bathroom surfaces, including the bathtub, tiles, basin, taps, and shower panels. Unlike commercial bathroom sprays, the paste adheres well to surfaces, such as the bathtub and tile grout, so you can clean them more effectively.

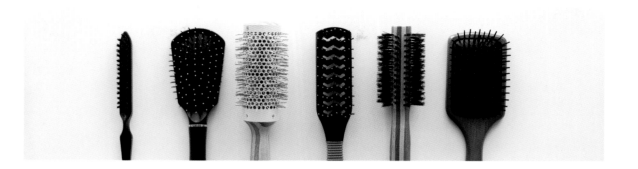

HAIRBRUSHES, COMBS, MAKEUP BRUSHES

Once a month, these need cleaning. Mix 4 tbsp bicarbonate of soda in 1 litre (2 pints) hot water, and add 10 drops **tea tree essential oil**. Soak your combs, hairbrushes, and makeup brushes and sponges in the solution for 1 hour. If they are quite messy, rub the brushes and combs against each other to remove all the hair from them. Rinse them in cold water.

PIPES

Is water draining away too slowly, and are nasty smells coming up from the basin? If so, it is time to do something about your pipes. Mix 200 g (7 oz) table salt with 200 g (7 oz) bicarbonate of soda, and pour this down your sink or wash basin, or other pipes. Then pour down 1 glass of warmed white vinegar (that will foam, so don't breathe in the vapour), and leave this for a night. The next day, pour down a solution of 10 drops **lemon essential oil** mixed with 1 litre (2 pints) boiling water.

SHOWERHEADS

Pour 500 ml (17 fl oz) white vinegar into a plastic bag, and add 10 drops **lemon essential oil**. Attach the bag to the showerhead (tie the handles round it), then gently turn on the tap to fill the bag with hot water, but not so much that it overflows. The idea is to let the showerhead soak in the mixture, so that the vinegar can dislodge the limescale, and the lemon essential oil can clean the head. Leave it on for a minimum of 2 hours.

SHOWER CURTAINS

Mildew loves shower curtains. It mixes with soap residue and can get so bad that you simply have to throw the shower curtain away. But you can give the curtain new life with this clever solution. Pour 5 tbsp sodium bicarbonate and 10 drops **tea tree essential oil** into 1 litre (2 pints) hot water. Soak a clean sponge in the mixture, then rub the affected areas vigorously. Rinse with luke-warm water.

CLEAN TAPS

Mix 25 g (⅘ oz) powdered white clay with 150 ml (5 fl oz) 'Miracle' laundry detergent (page 104), and 30 drops **lemon essential oil**. Pour this into a metal box, and let it dry out uncovered for a week. Once it has solidified, the block of clay is ready for use. Moisten a sponge, rub it on the clay block, and polish your taps. Leave the metal box open for while immediately after use, so that the block can dry out again.

THE SMALLEST ROOM

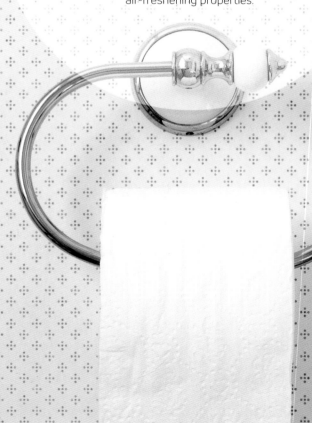

MIRACLE
TOILET SPRAY

Ingredients:
500 ml (17 fl oz) white vinegar,
15 drops **lemon essential oil**

Pour the ingredients into a 500 ml (17 fl oz) spray bottle,
then shake well to mix. The two make a great team;
the white vinegar gets rid of areas of limescale, where
bacteria and smells accumulate, and the **lemon essential oil**
gets behind it, using its antiseptic, antibacterial,
air-freshening properties.

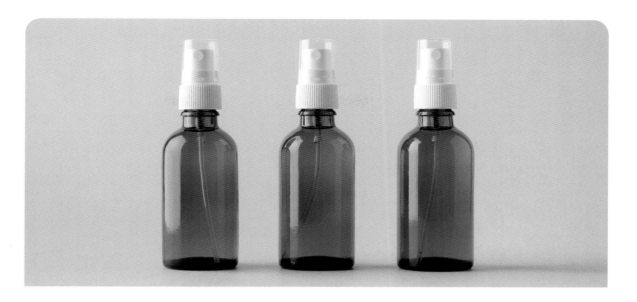

AIR FRESHENER

Where do you want to be – in the Alps or Provence? You get to decide what sort of environment you'd like to create with this recipe – through your choice of **lavender, rosemary, peppermint,** or **lemon essential oil.** Dilute ½ tsp of your chosen essential oil in 2 tbsp Isopropyl alcohol 70%. Pour the mixture into a 300 ml (10 fl oz) spray bottle, add 200 ml (6¾ fl oz) spring water, and shake well to mix it. Leave the bottle on hand for anyone using the facilities, but up high, out of reach of little ones.

TOILET LIMESCALE REMOVER

This is perhaps the cleverest of our household products, as it works all by itself. Simply spray around the edge of the toilet bowl each day, and that's it. Pour 1 glass of white vinegar, 2 tbsp black liquid soap, ½ glass of bicarbonate of soda, and 6 drops **rosemary cineole essential oil** into a spray bottle. Shake well each time before using it.

DISINFECTING WIPES

Mix 100 ml (3⅓ fl oz) white vinegar, 1 tbsp washing-up liquid, and 100 ml (3⅓ fl oz) spring water in a bowl. Add 5 drops **tea tree essential oil** and 5 drops **lemon essential oil,** and stir well until the mixture is smooth. Get some thick kitchen roll, take off 50 pieces, then fold each one in two. Place these clean 'wipes' in a sealable plastic bag (or box), and pour the essential oil mixture over them. Wait for 2 hours before using them. Periodically, turn the bag (or box) upside down so that the wipes remain impregnated with the essential oil fragrance. Throw the wipes away after use.

DOOR HANDLES

Find an old glove made of cotton, wool, or any absorbent material. Pour 2 drops **lemon essential oil** onto the palm of the glove and 2 drops on the fingers. Clean the door handles regularly with this disinfecting glove.

WARDROBES

MIRACLE
AIR FRESHENER
Ingredients:
40 drops **lemon essential oil**
150 ml (5 fl oz) white vinegar
250 ml (8½ fl oz) water

Pour the **lemon essential oil** and vinegar into a clean spray bottle, and shake well. Spray your 'miracle' freshener all around the wardrobe, on every shelf, rack, and hanging rail. Before closing the wardrobe door, wipe the bottom of the door with a cloth soaked in the solution. The next person who opens it will be greeted with a refreshing lemon fragrance.

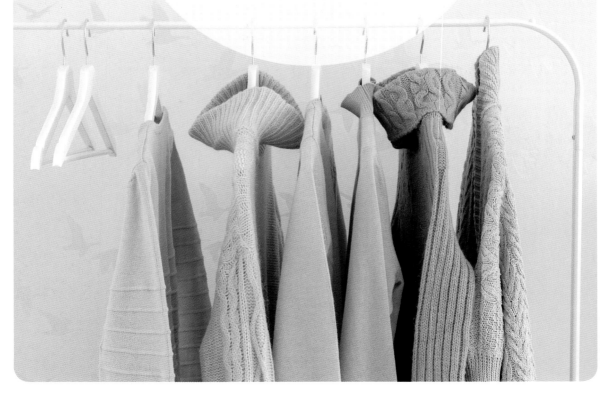

SHOE DEODORIZER

Add 5 drops **lavender essential oil** to 1 tbsp bicarbonate of soda, then pour the mixture into one sock. Do the same thing with the other sock. Place the socks inside your shoes. Just one night with bicarbonate, an avid consumer of bad smells, and the cleansing lavender essential oil will refresh your shoes. And the sweet-smelling socks will do no harm, so you can leave them in place for as long as you like.

CLOTHES FRESHENER

Pour 1 litre (2 pints) water into a saucepan, and bring to the boil. Take the pan off the heat, add 10 drops **lavender essential oil**, then stir. Put the item that needs freshening on a hanger, and hang it about 10 cm (4 in) – or higher, if the fabric is delicate – above the steaming saucepan. The steam will rise, enveloping the item, and giving it the fragrance of lavender, just as if it had been newly cleaned.

LITTLE PERFUME SACHET

Cut out a circle of fabric about 25 cm (10 in) in diameter. Pour 2 drops **lavender essential oil** onto a round cotton wool pad, and place it in the middle of the fabric circle. Then pour 2 tbsp lavender flowers (fresh or dried) onto the cotton wool pad. Make a little bag out of the piece of fabric, by pulling up the sides, then securing it with ribbon, raffia, or thread. Slip the sachet into a drawer, or hook it onto a hanger.

SPORTS BAG

Teams of bacteria are, almost certainly, playing their own games inside that bag. If the bag is machine washable, launder it at least once a month, adding 10 drops **tea tree essential oil** diluted in 1 glass of white vinegar to the fabric conditioner compartment. If you can't put it in the washing machine, spray it with 'Miracle' air freshener after each sports session.

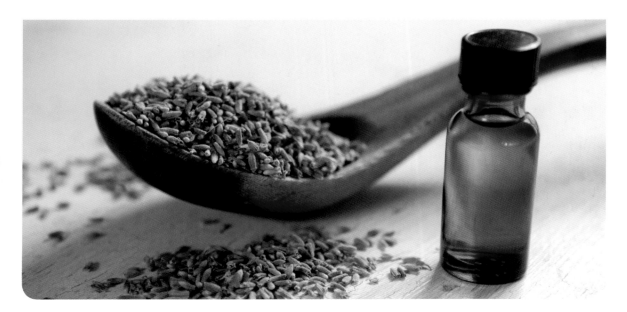

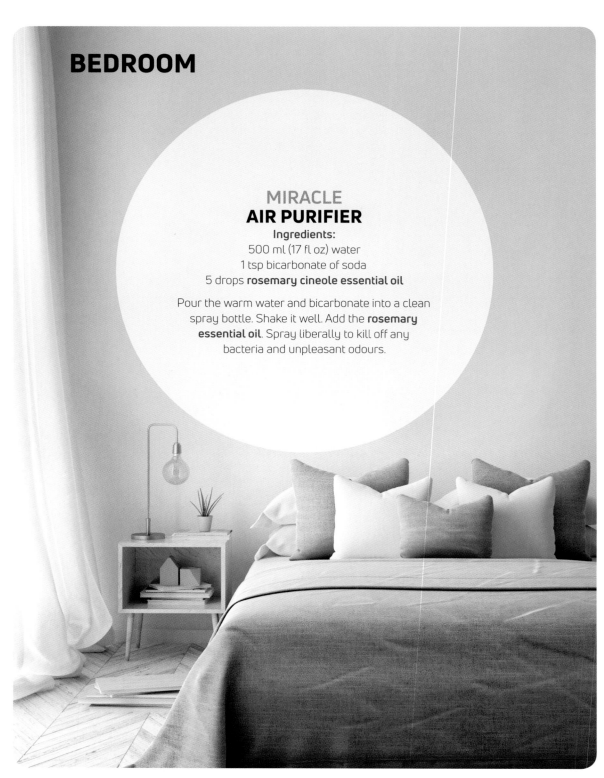

BEDROOM

MIRACLE
AIR PURIFIER
Ingredients:
500 ml (17 fl oz) water
1 tsp bicarbonate of soda
5 drops **rosemary cineole essential oil**

Pour the warm water and bicarbonate into a clean spray bottle. Shake it well. Add the **rosemary essential oil**. Spray liberally to kill off any bacteria and unpleasant odours.

GERM-FREE BEDCLOTHES – ANTI-FLU SPECIALIST

To avoid any risk of infection or germs spread by bedclothes, prepare this disinfecting solution by mixing 2 ml **lemon essential oil** with 1 ml **rosemary cineole essential oil**, and use it as follows. Soak the sheets, pillowcases, and nightclothes in warm water plus 10 drops of the essential oil solution for half an hour. Then launder them in the usual way, but add 4 to 5 drops of the solution to the fabric conditioner compartment. If washing by hand, add only 2 drops of the solution to the last rinse.

SHEETS

Given the number of dust mites that can lodge in sheets and the studies that show the horrible microbes that may be there, it's time to find a solution.

- Change your sheets once a week. Wash them in very hot water, and add 6 drops **tea tree essential oil** mixed with 1 glass of white vinegar to the fabric conditioner compartment of your washing machine.
- Pour 6 drops **lemon essential oil** onto a clean cloth, and put it into your tumble dryer with your sheets.
- Iron your sheets after spraying them with a solution of 500 ml (17 fl oz) de-ionized water and 4 drops **lavender essential oil**. Shake the spray bottle well before use.

ANTI-MITE MATTRESS

If it's war they're after, the fight is on. Every month, get out a spray-gun filled with a mixture of fresh lemon juice, 1 tbsp **lavender essential oil** and 750 ml (1½ pints) water. First thing in the morning, surprise the bugs by spraying each side of the mattress, then wait until evening before remaking the bed.

SLEEP-INDUCING PILLOWS

One small action can gain you a full night's sleep. Pour 2 drops **lavender essential oil** onto each pillow before going to bed.

ST VALENTINE'S SPECIAL

ROSE-SCENTED STATIONERY FROM THE HEART Slip 10 sheets of writing paper into a freezer bag with a zip fastener. Pour 10 drops **damask rose essential oil** onto a piece of fabric, folded several times, so that the oil will not touch the paper when you put the fabric into the plastic bag. Zip it up, and leave for 48 hours to let the essential oil get to work.

MINT CHOCOLATE BONBONS FOR SHARED BATHS Melt 4 tbsp cocoa butter, using the bain-marie method (see page 32). Add 2 tbsp sweet almond carrier oil, and keep stirring. Take the pan off the heat, and stir in 20 drops **peppermint essential oil**, mixing well. Pour the preparation into heart-shaped moulds, then freeze for 3 hours. Take the hearts out of their moulds, and wrap in different-coloured tissue papers. When the magic moment arrives, unwrap two, and throw them in the bath; they will melt, giving off a sweet scent.

CHILD'S BEDROOM

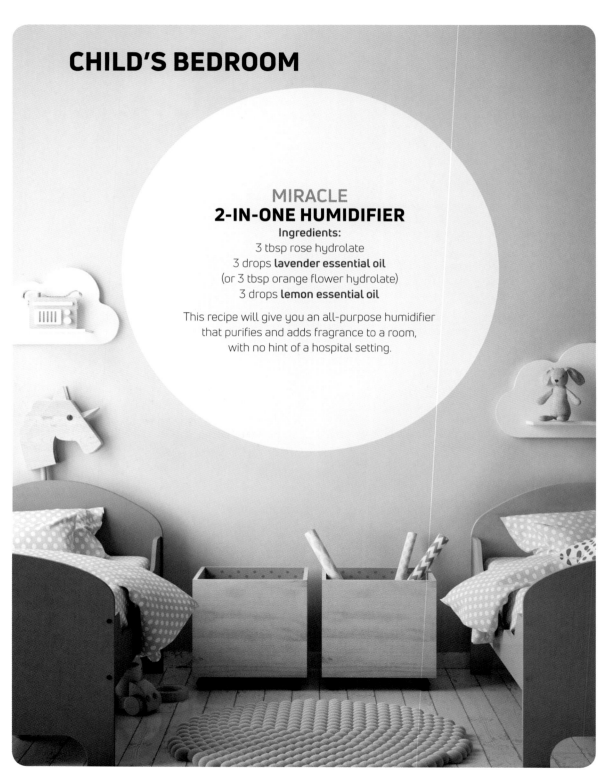

MIRACLE
2-IN-ONE HUMIDIFIER
Ingredients:
3 tbsp rose hydrolate
3 drops **lavender essential oil**
(or 3 tbsp orange flower hydrolate)
3 drops **lemon essential oil**

This recipe will give you an all-purpose humidifier
that purifies and adds fragrance to a room,
with no hint of a hospital setting.

FOR GIRLS

Mix together 3 tbsp rose hydrolate and 3 drops **lavender essential oil** in a bowl. Leave the bowl on the radiator all night.

FOR BOYS

Mix together 3 tbsp orange flower hydrolate and 3 drops **lemon essential oil** in a bowl. Place the bowl on a radiator and leave it there all night.

CLEANSING DIFFUSION

In the evening, pour 10 drops **lavender essential oil** into the diffuser, and diffuse for 1 hour before the child goes to bed.

TOYS

You really cannot wash toys, especially not a beloved teddy or comforter, in suspect detergents, knowing that sooner or later they'll be going into your baby's mouth. Instead, fill a bathtub with hot water, add 1 glass of Marseille soap flakes, 1 glass of white vinegar, and 10 drops **lemon essential oil**. Stir with your hand to mix the ingredients. Allow the toys to soak in the solution for around 30 minutes, then rinse them off with a lot of water.

MATTRESS

Little accidents will quickly mark a mattress. Bicarbonate of soda, with its supreme ability to soak up moisture and consume odours, will act on such stains in a flash. Sprinkle the bicarbonate liberally over the mattress, even if it isn't stained; if it is, rub the stains with a damp cloth dipped in bicarbonate. Leave for 2 hours, then carefully vacuum the mattress. For final antibacterial protection, spray a few drops **lavender essential oil** on the mattress.

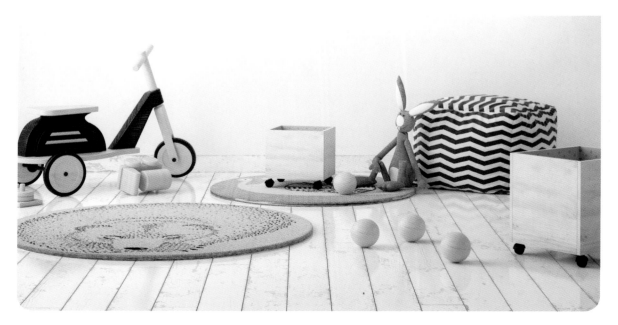

LIVING ROOM

MIRACLE
CARPET REVIVER
Ingredients:
300 ml (10 fl oz) white vinegar
3 tbsp bicarbonate of soda
10 drops **lavender essential oil**
150 ml (5 fl oz) super-effective washing-up liquid (see page 101)

- Mix the ingredients in a 500 ml (17 fl oz) spray bottle. Wait until the mixture froths when the vinegar comes into contact with the bicarbonate. It can take you by surprise; don't inhale it.
- Test the solution on a corner of the carpet that can't be seen to ensure that it doesn't react with the fabric; leave it for 2 hours.
- Vacuum the whole area of the carpet you wish to clean, then lightly spray the surface with the solution. Using a clean cloth, work on the stains, adding a little of the solution but not too much. Go round each one. Leave as long as possible before walking on it; the drier the carpet or rug, the better the result.

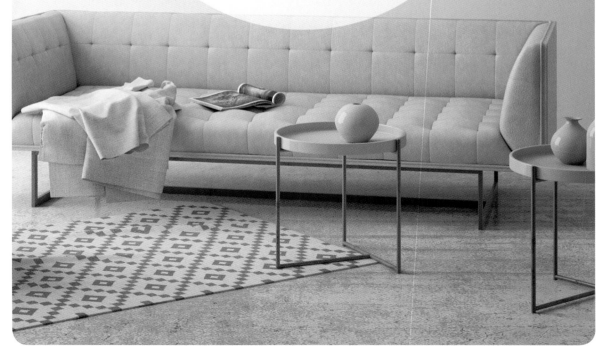

FRAGRANT VACUUMING

Pour 10 drops **lavender essential oil** onto a cotton wool ball, place it on the floor, and vacuum it up. The fragrance of the lavender will replace the smell of compacted dust in your machine every time you use it. Using dried or fresh lavender works just as well. Scatter some lavender on the floor and vacuum it up.

CLEAN A LEATHER WATCHSTRAP

How can a leather watchstrap smell so bad after only two months' wear? Again, it's a question of bacteria. They love areas that are warm and moist from perspiration and get into the leather itself. Mix 2 drops **lemon essential oil** with 1 tsp body lotion (a moisturizer or cleanser), pour a little onto a cotton wool pad, and clean the inside of the watchstrap.

FRESH LEMON ASHTRAY

At last, a useful little idea to avoid cleaning ashtrays while holding your nose. The smell of ash, mixed with washing-up liquid, diffused by hot water – horrible! Pour enough salt into the ashtray to cover its base. Then add 2 drops **lemon essential oil**. Roll up some kitchen roll into a ball, rub the ashtray with it, then rinse it in hot water.

PINE OIL POLISH

It's no. 1 of our top five homely smells; polish makes us think of comfort and cleanliness. Our favourite essential oils have all the necessary properties to help you prepare a furniture wax, while turpentine, the volatile oil distilled from pine resin, will discourage infestation.

Put a 250 g (9 oz) block of beeswax into a covered heat-proof jam jar and melt it using the bain-marie method (see page 32). When the wax has melted, take the pan off the heat and place it outside (on a balcony or in the garden) or in a well-ventilated room. Pour 250 ml (8½ fl oz) turpentine into the jar (still steeped in hot water in the bain-marie) and beat continuously. Leave the wax to cool, then add 10 drops **lavender essential oil** and 10 drops **lemon essential oil**, and continue beating the mixture. After using it to wax your furniture and make it shine, seal the jar tightly.

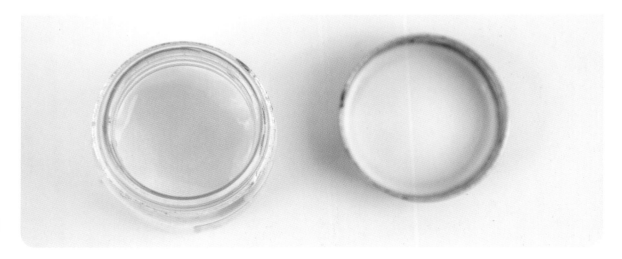

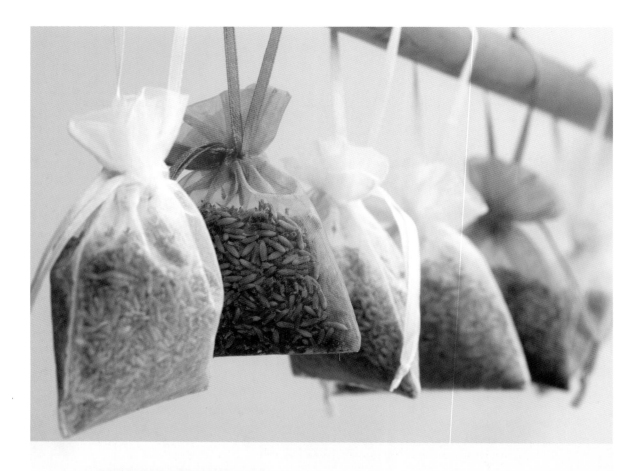

SCENTED SACHETS

Cut out a piece of fabric 10 x 5 cm (4 x 2 in) and fold it in two, with the right sides together. Sew up three sides (the two lengths and one width) ½ cm from the edge. Turn the right sides out and iron the sachet. Fill it about three-quarters full with the dried-flower or petal mixture you have chosen. Cut off a 16 cm (6 in) piece of ribbon or cord, and wrap it three times around the open end of your sachet, closing it with a double knot. Try making sachets with each of the fragrant fillings below, placing them in a pretty glass bowl, or a decorative sweet or biscuit tin.

THREE AROMATIC FILLINGS

Fragrant meadow sachet
1 handful of lavender flowers + 2 drops **lavender essential oil**

Fragrant garden sachet
1 handful of rosebuds + 2 drops **damask rose essential oil.**

Fragrant window-box sachet
1 handful of chopped verbena leaves + 2 drops **peppermint essential oil.**

AIR FRESHENER

Mix 200 ml (6¾ fl oz) water, 200 ml (6¾ fl oz) Isopropyl alcohol 60%, and 30 drops **lavender essential oil** in a spray bottle. Shake before each use, and spray every morning after airing the room.

QUICK POT-POURRI

Take 2 limes and 3 clementines (organic if possible), and cut each of them in half. Stick 3 cloves in each of the halves. Place them in a pretty dish or in an empty fish bowl, then pour in 10 drops **lemon essential oil**. Put your pot-pourri close to a heat source, such as a fireplace, radiator, or in sunlight.

VITAMIN-RICH WINDOW CLEANER

Pour 250 ml (8½ fl oz) de-ionized water and 150 ml (5 fl oz) white vinegar into a spray bottle, and mix. Add 5 drops **lemon essential oil**, and shake well. Use as you would a commercial window cleaning product, applying it with a clean cloth or piece of kitchen roll. This clever cleaning formula will ensure that your windows are clean and bacteria free, and the glass will attract less dust.

RUG CLEANER

Crumbs, animal hair, bits of everything brought in from outside – rugs are a haven for bacteria. A dry shampoo with essential oils will clean all that up in a couple of hours. Pour 200 g (7 oz) bicarbonate of soda and 40 drops **tea tree essential oil** into a plastic container with a lid. Close the container, shake it, then leave for 8 hours, so that the bicarbonate can absorb the essential oil. Spread the powder all over the rug; you can fold it up and walk on it, if you're really keen, to ensure the mixture has fully penetrated the fibres. Like a regular dry shampoo, the bicarbonate will absorb grease and smells, while the essential oil will kill off bacteria. Leave it on for 4 hours, then vacuum the rug.

SPIDER DETERRENT

You've flushed them out of their favourite haunts, such as the bathroom, and ceiling corners. Now you need to add 2 drops **lavender essential oil** to cotton wool balls, then place them strategically in your home. If the mere sight of a spider frightens you, use a spray; pour 1 tsp **lavender essential oil** into a spray bottle and fill it up with Isopropyl alcohol 70% (available from pharmacies and online).

KEEP FLIES AWAY

Luckily for us, the fragrance of lavender deters flies. Pour 200 ml (6¾ fl oz) water into a spray bottle, and add 10 drops **lavender essential oil**. Shake well, then spray the tops and edges of your windows and doors. The flies will stay away.

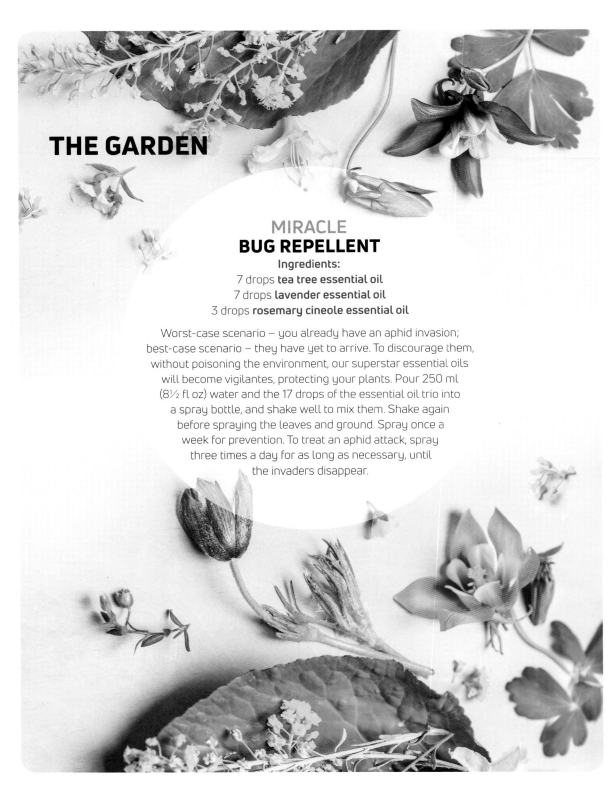

THE GARDEN

MIRACLE
BUG REPELLENT

Ingredients:

7 drops **tea tree essential oil**

7 drops **lavender essential oil**

3 drops **rosemary cineole essential oil**

Worst-case scenario – you already have an aphid invasion; best-case scenario – they have yet to arrive. To discourage them, without poisoning the environment, our superstar essential oils will become vigilantes, protecting your plants. Pour 250 ml (8½ fl oz) water and the 17 drops of the essential oil trio into a spray bottle, and shake well to mix them. Shake again before spraying the leaves and ground. Spray once a week for prevention. To treat an aphid attack, spray three times a day for as long as necessary, until the invaders disappear.

DISCOURAGE ANTS

Ants are no joke. A column of them can clear out your food cupboards. Arm yourself with a weapon that will get rid of them. Pour 250 ml (8½ fl oz) Isopropyl alcohol 40% into a spray bottle, and add 5 drops **lavender essential oil** and 10 drops **peppermint essential oil**, then shake well. Spray this mixture several times a day for several days along the route the ants use.

BANISH MOSQUITOES

Mosquitoes don't like **lavender** or **peppermin**t, so you can keep them away with a cocktail of the two essential oils. Pour equal parts into a diffuser, and let it work for 20 minutes.

REFRESH WOODEN FURNITURE

Rain has attacked the shine on your garden dining furniture, and the sun has dried out the wood. A little vitamin-rich treatment can restore it. Squeeze the juice of a fresh lemon into a bowl, and add 1 tsp olive oil and 5 drops **lemon essential oil**, then mix. Soak a cloth in the solution, and wipe the garden table in the direction of the wood grain. Finish by rubbing it with a duster to make it shine. If you like the result, have a go at the chairs.

A WELCOMING DOORMAT

It's no secret; if you want a doormat that keeps dirt out of the house, you have to look after it. Pour 200 g (7 oz) bicarbonate of soda into a bowl, then add 20 drops **rosemary cineole essential oil**, and mix. Sprinkle the doormat with the mixture, and wipe your feet on it to help the mixture penetrate the fibres. Leave it to work for 20 minutes. Then, using a hard brush, give it a vigorous brushing, and, lastly, vacuum the mat to finish the job.

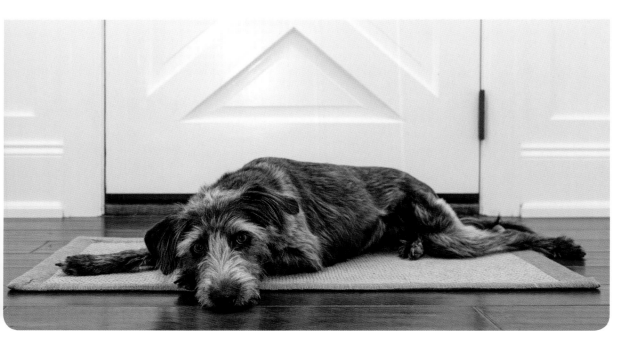

IMPROVE YOUR PETS' LIVES

MIRACLE
TICK AND FLEA
TREATMENT

Ingredients (for dogs):

2 drops **lavender essential oil**

2 drops **peppermint essential oil**

2–4 tsp olive oil

For dogs: Combine the essential oils, and dilute with olive oil according to your pet's size – 2 tsp for large dogs and up to 4 tsp for smaller dogs. Mix well, then rub the solution onto your pet's hair, being careful to avoid the eyes, nose, mouth, and genitals. Alternatively, put a few drops of the solution on the outside of a bandana or collar made of absorbent cloth.

For cats: Cats cannot tolerate essential oils, so try spritzing a gentler lavender hydrolate onto your cat's fur.

Caution: Neither dogs or cats should ingest essential oils, as they can cause a dangerous reaction. Don't apply essential oils or hydrolates if your pet objects to the smell.

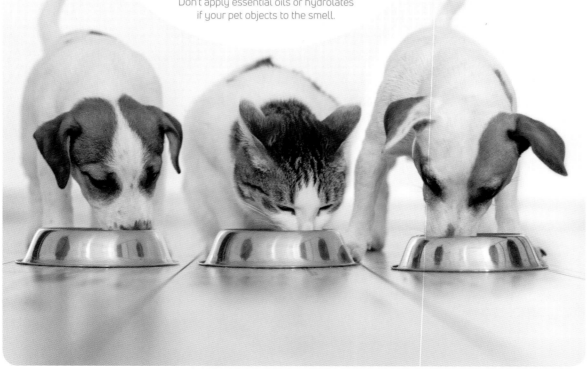

TOYS, DISHES, CAGES – ALL IN THE BATH

All your pet's toys and accessories will emerge clean and odourless from this bath. Depending on how many you need to wash, fill up a bowl or bathtub with hot water. Pour in 4 tbsp bicarbonate of soda and 5 drops **tea tree essential oil**. Soak everything for half an hour, then rinse in clear water.

FIRST AID

If your dog has a cut or a skin irritation, don't worry. **Lavender essential oil** can help and will also relieve skin irritations. In a spray bottle, mix up to 30 drops of essential oil with one cup of water (fewer drops for smaller dogs). A few drops of lavender essential oil can also be combined with 1 tsp olive oil and used topically on sores or wounds. For a cat, try a good quality lavender hydrolate, as cats can be highly sensitive to essential oils.

DOG-PROOF YOUR PLANTS

You've only just unwrapped your new garden plant, and your dog is there, preparing to baptize it. Pour 500 ml (17 fl oz) water and 20 drops **lavender essential oil** into a spray bottle. Shake it, then spray the earth and the plant pot your dog is targeting.

IF IT'S TOO LATE ...

Is he getting his own back or is it an accident? Your dog has marked his territory with a smell that is instantly recognizable and difficult to remove. And it's been there a while. Pour 2 tsp bicarbonate of soda into a medium-sized bowl, and then pour in white vinegar until it is about three-quarters full (you need some space as it momentarily froths up.) Add 3 drops **lavender essential oil**, and mix. Soak a clean cloth in the solution, and rub the affected areas. Rinse with warm water. When it is dry, vacuum if necessary to remove any of the bicarbonate residue.

PET GROOMING

Pets are also entitled to fragrant hair care. Let your dog sniff a few essential oil fragrances, then add a few drops of his favourite to a regular shampoo. Similarly, consult your cat about hydrolates, then spray a little of her preferred one on her fur, and comb through.

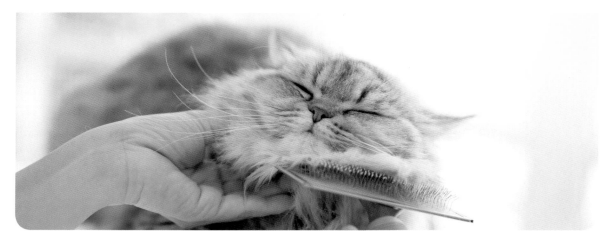

10 BONUS ESSENTIAL OILS

Now you've discovered the powerful properties of our six favourite, indispensable essential oils, you may like to explore further. Here are ten of the most popular, together with their key properties and their primary uses. All are readily available from high street stores specializing in natural herbal products, or online.

BERGAMOT *Citrus bergamia*
Key properties: antibiotic, analgesic, skin-healing, deodorant, sedative, antidepressant
Can be used for: relieving pain, reducing fever, alleviating digestive problems, clearing chest congestion.

EUCALYPTUS *Eucalyptus globulus*
Key properties: cleansing, anti-inflammatory, decongestant, antibacterial
Can be used for: decongesting the nose and sinuses, controlling coughing, relieving sore throats, easing joint and muscle pain.

FRANKINCENSE *Boswellia carterii*
Key properties: antiseptic, astringent, antimicrobial, boosts immune system
Can be used for: relieving stress and anxiety, treating bronchitis and extreme coughing, healing and minimizing scars and stretch marks.

GINGER *Zingiber officinale*
Key properties: anti-emetic, digestive aid, analgesic, antiseptic, carminative, stimulant
Can be used for: relieving nausea, enhancing concentration, mood-boosting, reducing stress, anxiety, and fatigue.

JASMINE *Jasminum grandiflorum*
Key properties: antidepressant, antiseptic, aphrodisiac, antispasmodic, sedative
Can be used for: relieving depression, treating dry or sensitive skin, alleviating exhaustion, easing labour pains.

MANDARIN *Citrus reticulata*
Key properties: antiseptic, antispasmodic, digestive, nervous relaxant, sedative, tonic
Can be used for: treating acne and other skin conditions, healing scars, relieving insomnia, reducing stress, minimizing wrinkles.

Can be used for: relieving congestion, bronchitis, sore throats and coughs, reducing flatulence, soothing mouth and gum disorders.

NEROLI *Citrus aurantium*
Key properties: antidepresssant, antiseptic, aphrodisiac, skin-healing, digestive, tonic
Can be used for: relieving depression and insomnia, treating skin problems (including scars, stretch marks, and mature skin).

PINE *Pinus sylvestris*
Key properties: antibacterial, decongestant, diuretic, stimulant, anitviral, antifungal
Can be used for: protecting against infection, optimizing blood circulation, easing stiff muscles.

SANDALWOOD *Santalum album*
Key properties: astringent, antiseptic, antiviral, anti-inflammatory, expectorant
Can be used for: treating bronchitis and laryngitis, easing stress and depression, relieving urinary tract infections, skin-healing.

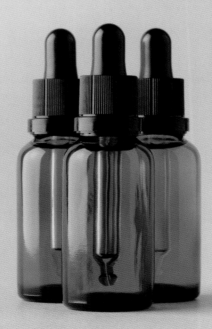

INDEX

PICTURE CREDITS

Front Cover (left to right)
spline_x, MaraZe, Rtstudio, oxygen_8, Nattika, DragonPhotos, saiko3p/ShutterStockphoto.Inc
Back Cover Lina Keil/ShutterStockphoto.Inc

ShutterStockphoto.Inc 2-3 Patricia Chumillas; 4 P Maxwell Photography; 7 matka_Wariatka; 9 Shablon; 10 Image Point Fr; 11 (left to right) spline_x, MaraZe, Rtstudio, Nattika, DragonPhotos, saiko3p; 12 spline_x; 13 (plant) Lina Keil; 13 (bottle) (oxygen_8); 14 saiko3p; 15 (plant) lena_nikolaeva; 15 (bottle) (oxygen_8); 16 DragonPhotos; 17 (plant) Lina Keil; 17 (bottle) (oxygen_8); 18 Varts; 19 (plant) aniana; 19 (bottle) (oxygen_8); 20 Igor Dutina; 21 (plant) Morphart Creation; 21 (bottle) (oxygen_8); 22 Rtstudio; 23 (plant) umiko; 23 (bottle) (oxygen_8); 24-5 Shablon; 26-7 Alena Ozerova; 28 Leonid and Anna Dedukh; 29 Comaniciu Dan; 31 Image Point Fr; 33 Vladimir Gjorgiev; 34 onair; 34-5 Sehenswerk; 36-7 Alliance; 38 Stacey Newman; 39 Elle1; 40 Lopolo; 41 kariphoto; 43 Guschenkova; 45 UfaBizPhoto; 46 Mal2TH; 47 Rido; 48 Jacob Lund; 49 Africa Studio; 50 StudioPhotoDFlorez; 51 sukiyaki; 52 FotoDuets; 53 Dmitrii Ivanov; 55 Africa Studio; 56 takayuki; 57 Shablon; 58 Alena Ozerova; 61 nelen; 65 Daniel_Dash; 67 Milan Ilic Photographer; 69 Roman Samborskyi; 70 Nina Buday; 71t P Maxwell Photography; 71b puhhha; 72 B-D-S Piotr Marcinski; 73 rebvt; 74-5 Aleshyn_Andrei; 76 George Rudy; 77t Claudio Divizia; 77b makalex69; 78 Africa Studio; 79, 80 Image Point Fr; 81 VICUSCHKA; 83 Demkat; 84 paulaphoto; 85 Africa Studio; 86 Syda Productions; 87 Image Point Fr; 88 Irina Bg; 89 Layland Masuda; 90 Image Point Fr; 91 Jason Squyres; 92, 94 Image Point Fr; 95 Ljupco Smokovski; 96 Image Point Fr; 98-9 Alena Ozerova; 100 Demkat; 103 Didecs; 104 Yuganov Konstantin; 105 Olga Pink; 106 Demkat; 107 Syda Productions; 109 Shablon; 110 Ira Shpiller; 111 Mona Makela; 112, 114, 115, 116 mtlapcevic; 117 BoBoMuMu; 118 Gyorgy Barna; 120 VICUSCHKA; 121 Susan Schmitz; 122 Gladskikh Tatiana; 123 ANURAK PONGPATIMET 125 Shablon

iStockphoto 63 GlobalStock; 108 bigworld

ACKNOWLEDGEMENTS

Eddison Books Limited
Managing Director **Lisa Dyer**
Creative Consultant **Nick Eddison**
Managing Editor **Tessa Monina**
Translation **Rachel Warren Chadd**
Designed and edited by **Fogdog Creative** (www.fogdog.co.uk)
Proofreader **Marianne Taylor**
Indexer **Marie Lorimer**
Production **Sarah Rooney & Cara Clapham**